STUDENT WORKBOOK

FOR

LABORATORY PROCEDURES FOR MEDICAL OFFICE PERSONNEL

STUDENT WORKBOOK

FOR

LABORATORY PROCEDURES FOR MEDICAL OFFICE PERSONNEL

MARYANN WOODS, PhD, RN, CMA
Professor, Health Science Division
Director of Medical Assistant-Clinician Program
Fresno City College, Fresno, California
Member of California Certifying Board for Medical Assistants
Member of California Association of Medical Assistant Instructors

SAUNDERS
An Imprint of Elsevier

Saunders
An Imprint of Elsevier

The Curtis Center
Independence Square West
Philadelphia, Pennsylvania 19106-3399

Student Workbook for
Laboratory Procedures for Medical Office Personnel

ISBN-13: 978-0-7216-5276-4
ISBN-10: 0-7216-5276-X

Printed in the United States of America.

Last digit is the print number: 9 8 7 6 5

PREFACE

Student Workbook

for

Laboratory Procedures for Medical Office Personnel

This workbook was designed to ensure that the student has a positive learning experience. The exercises will add to the student's understanding as he or she experiences learning by doing. Each chapter contains vocabulary reinforcement, review questions, and critical thinking problems.

The workbook was designed to give the students "on the job" situations. In some instances, the student will need to use reference texts in addition to their textbook to obtain the correct answers. This was intentionally done to familiarize the student with the concept that all answers are not found in one book and that research is part of continuing education.

I sincerely hope that using this Student Workbook will provide a pleasurable learning experience to students and assist them in enlarging their scope of laboratory knowledge.

MaryAnn Woods, PhD, RN, CMA

Contributing Author: Lance Granum, LVN, CMA

TABLE of CONTENTS

UNIT I INTRODUCTION TO THE MEDICAL LABORATORY

CHAPTER 1 THE MEDICAL LABORATORY

MATCHING

Match the terms in the right column with the definitions in the left column by writing the letters in the blanks.

_____ 1. Laboratory medicine that studies blood serum for evidence of infection by evaluating antigen-antibody reactions in vitro.

_____ 2. Hidden or difficult to observe directly.

_____ 3. Analysis of purity or effectiveness of any biological substances including drugs.

_____ 4. The scientific study of poisons, their detection, effects, and methods of treatment for conditions they produce.

_____ 5. Study of cells and their formation.

a. Assay
b. Cytology
c. Occult
d. Serology
e. Toxicology

SHORT ANSWER

Answer the following questions:

6. List five skills that the assistant/phlebotomist must demonstrate before assuming responsibility in the laboratory.

____

____

____

____

____

7. Identify five types of nonhospital laboratory facilities.

_____________________ _____________________

_____________________ _____________________

____

8. In the microbiology section of the lab, major methods for analysis include the following:

____

____

9. List the section of the laboratory that would perform the following tests:

Blood glucose:________________________________

Occult blood:________________________________

Hematology:________________________________

BUN:________________________________

Fungus Antibody :________________________________

Culture and sensitivity:________________________________

CBC:________________________________

Chromosomal analysis:________________________________

VDRL:________________________________

Autopsy:________________________________

Rh antibody titer:________________________________

CRITICAL THINKING

Decide how you would handle the following situations, using the knowledge you have obtained in this chapter, combined with previously learned knowledge.

SITUATION #1

Jane Castic, CMA, is employed by a multi-care facility and works in the laboratory. Recently the facility hired Frank Souza as new laboratory assistant/phlebotomist. This individual has ten years of experience as a phlebotomist and appears to be very well qualified. One afternoon as you are running a series of urine reagent tests, you notice that Frank is completing a number of blood counts, posting the results on the requisition forms, and rubber stamping the signatures with the laboratory technologist's signature stamp. You ask him if he is allowed to enter the test results and stamp them without the tech verifying the results, and he tells you that he has been doing these tests for so many years that he is better at them than any tech and the doctors all know it. "Besides, if I get these tests done and in the mail, we'll all get out of here on time!"

1. What do you think Jane should do?

____

____

____

2. Is Frank allowed to enter test results without the lab tech verifying the results? Why?

____

____

3. If an error would occur and cause a patient harm, who do you think would be responsible?

____

____

SITUATION #2

You have read about the levels of expertise that are utilized within the laboratory and having completed Procedure 1, you have interviewed someone working in the laboratory. Using the accumulated knowledge, analyze your personal interests and answer the following questions.

1. What laboratory area do you feel you would feel comfortable working in? Why?

____

____

____

2. What area do you think would be the most difficult area to work in? Why?

____

____

____

3. How do you feel about employment opportunities within the laboratory area? Why?

____

____

____

CHAPTER 2 SAFETY IN THE LABORATORY

MATCHING

Match the terms in the right column with the definitions in the left column by writing the letters in the blanks.

Definitions	Terms
_____ 1. The production of pus and purulent matter.	a. Asymptomatic
_____ 2. The process by which certain cells surround, engulf, and digest microorganisms and cellular debris.	b. Benign
_____ 3. An interstitial collection of fluid.	c. Caustic
_____ 4. Without signs and symptoms.	d. Edema
_____ 5. Capable of boiling at a low temperature or evaporating quickly at room temperature.	e. Germicidal agent
_____ 6. Disease associated with toxins in the blood, blood poisoning.	f. Pathogens
_____ 7. Any substance that is destructive to living tissue.	g. Phagocytosis
_____ 8. Noncancerous, not life-threatening.	h. Septicemia
_____ 9. Any disease-producing agent or microorganism.	i. Suppuration
_____ 10. A drug that kills pathogenic microorganisms.	j. Volatile

SHORT ANSWER

Answer the following questions:

11. Identify the OSHA product warning labels pictured:

__________ __________ __________ __________

12. A mandatory laboratory safety rule is: *Do not eat, drink, or smoke in the lab area.* Why?

____

____

____

____

13. Without opening your textbook, trace the chain of infection.

____

____

____

____

14. List, in order, the four specific reactions an individual's body initiates when attempting to destroy the invading pathogenic organism.

____

____

____

____

15. Outline the five types of hepatitis and list the effects of each type.

____

____

____

____

____

16. OSHA standards require that every lab have a written plan that includes specific health and safety measures that must be taken to minimize the risk of exposure. Identify these five control areas and include two examples for each control area.

____

____

____

____

CRITICAL THINKING

Decide how you would handle the following situations, using the knowledge you have obtained in this chapter, combined with previously learned knowledge.

SITUATION #1

You notice that in the office you work, many of the employees, including the physician, do not wash their hands before putting on gloves. You ask several fellow employees about the need to follow OSHA guidelines regarding handwashing and their comments are "since the doctor doesn't wash his or her hands, why should we? You really feel that something needs to be done to correct the situation.

1. How might this situation be handled?

____

____

____

2. Would you consider reporting this to any of those listed below? Why?

OSHA _______________

Insurance carrier _______________

The patients _______________

AMA _______________

3. Could this be reason to call a mandatory staff conference? Why?

____

____

SITUATION #2

Va Xiong has been hired by the Almondwood Clinic to work as a phlebotomist. In her orientation, she is asked if she has been immunized for hepatitis. She says that she has not and then she is informed that she must be immunized in order to work as a phlebotomist. Va has been told by friends that this immunization is very painful and that she may get liver disease as a result of the shots. She also has been told that the immunization is very expensive, and Va knows that she cannot afford the immunization. The clinic manager tells Va that she is to report for work next week on Monday and that she will be given the first injection of the hepatitis series on that day. Va goes home and discusses the immunization with her family and on Friday she calls the clinic manager and tells her that she has decided to refuse the position.

1. Why do you think Va refused the employment?

____

____

2. What information could have been given to Va at the interview that might have changed the outcome?

____

____

____

If you were the clinic manager, how would you have handled Va's phone call on Friday?

____

____

____

CHAPTER 3 QUALITY ASSURANCE/QUALITY CONTROL

MATCHING

Match the terms in the right column with the definitions in the left column by writing the letters in the blanks.

_____ 1. The range of test values expected for a designated population of individuals.

_____ 2. The testing and adjustment of test systems to provide a known relations between the measurement response and the substance value measured by the test.

_____ 3. The range of test values over which the relationship between the testing instrument, kit, or system's measurement response has been shown to be valid.

_____ 4. An individual authorized under state law to order tests or receive test results.

_____ 5. A method for obtaining laboratory test results that involves performing a series of steps by hand or by personal physical means.

a. Calibration

b. Authorized person

c. Manual testing

d. Reference value

e. Reportable range

SHORT ANSWER

Answer the following questions:

6. Explain the difference between quality assurance and quality control.

____

____

____

7. Compare the testing done in the POL with the testing complexity of the commercial laboratory.

____

____

____

8. List the six areas of preparation for inspection of a POL.

____

____

CRITICAL THINKING

Decide how you would handle the following situations, using the knowledge you have obtained in this chapter, combined with previously learned knowledge.

SITUATION #1

Design a documentation system that includes all steps taken in performing a urinary pregnancy detection test. Your documentation might include the physician's order, specimen collection, testing procedure, quality control measures, instrument and reagent maintenance, and reporting of test results. The sample procedure is in Chapter 9 of your textbook

SITUATION #2

Using an assigned section of the laboratory supply cabinets at school or in your training site, check all expiration dates. Remove all supplies that have expired and arrange the remaining supplies according to date, the oldest at the front and the newest at the back. Keep an inventory list of each item in the cabinet. Check the procedure manual for the procedures to be followed when destroying or discarding expired supplies. Document the number of or the amount of each expired item, the method of destruction, and who witnessed the destruction. Generate any report forms needed. Be sure that all the necessary information is included before signing the report.

1. What supplies did you inventory?

2. Identify the supplies that had expired.

3. What did you do with each of the expired supplies?

CHAPTER 4 THE MICROSCOPE

MATCHING

Match the terms in the right column with the definitions in the left column by writing the letters in the blanks.

_____ 1. A deposit of relatively insoluble material that settles to the bottom of a container of liquid.

_____ 2. Pertaining to organisms without a true nucleus.

_____ 3. Single-celled microscopic animals found in water and soil.

_____ 4. Primitive plants capable of producing their own food.

_____ 5. Pertaining to organisms with a true nucleus .

_____ 6. Unicellular microorganisms that do not have membrane-enclosed nuclei.

_____ 7. Microorganisms that live on decaying organic materials.

_____ 8. The study of the physical shape and size of a specimen.

_____ 9. A microscopic organism.

_____10. A nonnucleated immature red blood cell.

a. Algae
b. Bacteria
c. Eukaryotic
d. Fungi
e. Microbe
f. Morphology
g. Prokaryotic
h. Protozoa
i. Reticulocyte
j. Sediment

SHORT ANSWER

Answer the following questions:

11. The common laboratory microscope today is a

____

12. Darkfield microscopy is frequently used to study

____

13. Phase-contrast technique enables viewing of dense structures such as in

____

14. The detection of tubercle bacillus and mycobacterial identification is accomplished using the

____

15. Contrast the brightfield microscope with the electron microscope.

____

____

____

CRITICAL THINKING

Decide how you would handle the following situations, using the knowledge you have obtained in this chapter, combined with previously learned knowledge.

SITUATION #1

Look in the laboratory procedure manual and read the section on maintenance of the microscope. Write out a step-by-step procedure for performing this maintenance.

____

____

____

____

____

____

SITUATION #2

Why does the electron microscope take pictures for you to analyze instead of allowing you to view the specimen being analyzed? Research the information in the library and/or contact a local facility that has an electron microscope and prepare an analytical answer to this question.

____

____

____

____

____

____

CHAPTER 5 UNDERSTANDING LABORATORY MEASUREMENTS

MATCHING

Match the terms in the right column with the definitions in the left column by writing the letters in the blanks.

_____ 1. Metric prefix equal to 0.000 000 001 — a. Meter

_____ 2. SI Base unit for quantity — b. Liter

_____ 3. Metric abbreviation for one-tenth — c. Gram

_____ 4. Metric basic unit for length — d. Celsius

_____ 5. Metric basic unit for capacity — e. Milli

_____ 6. Metric prefix for 0.000 001 — f. Deci

_____ 7. SI base unit expressing temperature — g. Kelvin

_____ 8. Metric base unit for weight — h. Mole

_____ 9. Metric prefix for one-thousandth — i. Micro

_____10. Metric base unit for temperature — j. Nano

SHORT ANSWER

Answer the following questions:

11. Distance in the U.S. is measured in miles but in the metric system it would be measured in

____

12. For practical purposes, the milliliter is considered to be equivalent to

____

13. The International Bureau of Weights and Measurements is responsible for

____

14. Base units that are most frequently used in the clinical laboratory include

____

____

____

15. The metric system is based on 10 and its multiples thus, it can be expressed as

____

CRITICAL THINKING

Decide how you would handle the following situations, using the knowledge you have obtained in this chapter, combined with previously learned knowledge.

SITUATION #1

Complete the table using the basic unit of meter:

1000.0	= ______________________
100.0	= ______________________
10.0	= ______________________
1.0	= ______________________
0.1	= ______________________
0.01	= ______________________
0.001	= ______________________
0.0001	= ______________________
0.000 001	= ______________________
0.000 000 001	= ______________________

SITUATION #2

Identify five types of products that use metric system units. If you cannot think of five, go to a large supermarket and search the shelves until you locate five.

Product	**Metric System Unit Used**
______________________	______________________
______________________	______________________
______________________	______________________
______________________	______________________
______________________	______________________

UNIT II URINALYSIS

CHAPTER 6 INTRODUCTION TO THE URINARY SYSTEM AND URINALYSIS

MATCHING

Match the terms in the right column with the definitions in the left column by writing the letters in the blanks.

Definitions	Terms
______ 1. The process of urination.	a. Bowman's capsule
______ 2. The tube that carries urine from the kidney to the bladder.	b. Cortex
______ 3. Lying behind the peritoneum.	c. Hilum
______ 4. Basic unit of the kidney.	d. Glomerulus
______ 5. A cup-shaped membrane surrounding the glomerulus.	e. Medulla
______ 6. A notch in the medial border of the kidney.	f. Nephron
______ 7. The tube leading from the bladder to the urinary meatus.	g. Retroperitoneal
______ 8. The outer layer of the kidney.	h. Voiding
______ 9. A mass of capillaries located inside Bowman's capsule.	i. Ureter
______10. The inside portion of the kidney.	j. Urethra

SHORT ANSWER

Answer the following questions:

11. Identify the seven different observations made of urine by Ismail of Jurjani in 1000 A.D.

____

____

____

12. Describe the kidney.

____

____

____

13. Describe the nephron.

14. List the two purposes of the urinalysis procedure.

15. List the five procedural steps in the identification of the urinary specimen.

CRITICAL THINKING

Decide how you would handle the following situations, using the knowledge you have obtained in this chapter, combined with previously learned knowledge.

SITUATION #1

You are asked to run the physical and chemical tests on a fresh group of urinary samples. As you are setting up the equipment to run the tests, you notice that three of the samples have no patient identification on them. You ask the assistant that collected the samples if she can identify them and she comes in, apparently in an extreme hurry, puts labels on all three, and rushes out of the room. How would you proceed with your assignment. Justify your rationale.

SITUATION #2

Quality assurance is an important aspect in performing urinalysis. The use of daily controls is one important tool in lab performance. Describe how you think using control specimens will help to increase your self-confidence in performing the testing.

____

____

____

____

____

CHAPTER 7 COLLECTING THE URINE SPECIMENS

MATCHING

Match the terms in the right column with the definitions in the left column by writing the letters in the blanks.

	Definition	Term
_____	1. External opening of the urethra.	a. Analyte
_____	2. The cone-shaped enlargement at the end of the penis.	b. Aseptic
_____	3. The folds of tissue that form the external female genitalia.	c. Glans
_____	4. Capacity of a standard collection container.	d. Labia
_____	5. Specimen volume needed for urinalysis.	e. Sterile
_____	6. 24-hour urine collection testing.	f. 25 ml.
_____	7. Free of infection and/or infectious waste.	g. Addis test
_____	8. A substance or material being chemically analyzed.	h. Genitalia
_____	9. Free of all forms of microbial life.	i. 50 to 100 mL
_____	10. The reproductive organs.	j. Urinary meatus

SHORT ANSWER

Answer the following questions:

11. List and summarize the five guidelines for urine collection.

____

____

____

____

____

12. Write out what you would tell a patient who must collect a first morning specimen at home. Would there be a difference in your explanation depending on the sex of the patient?

____

____

____

____

____

13. When the patient delivers the 24-hour container to the office, how must you prepare the specimen for transport?

____

____

____

____

14. What is the range of normal volume of urine produced in adults, children, and infants?

____

____

____

15. List the items to be found in a commercial kit for a clean-catch specimen collection.

____

____

____

CRITICAL THINKING

Decide how you would handle the following situations, using the knowledge you have obtained in this chapter, combined with previously learned knowledge.

SITUATION #1

The lab request order reads test for *antibiotic sensitivity*. What type of a specimen would you need for this test? What type of collection material would you give Mrs. Snead, and how would you instruct her to obtain this specimen? If this was Mr. Snead how would you alter your instructions?

____

____

____

____

____

____

____

____

SITUATION #2

The urine sample for a patient that was seen at 5:00 p.m. yesterday is found in the collection cubicle this morning. The lab request reads *routine testing*. Can the urinalysis be run on this specimen? Justify your answer.

____

____

____

____

____

Procedure Evaluation Check-off

Use this form with your laboratory partner in practicing your procedures. Each student should have a minimum of two procedure evaluations done before requesting the instructor to observe his or her procedure technique for grading. **This form may be duplicated as often as needed**

Procedure Evaluation Form

NAME:____

PROCEDURE:____

Technique	Yes	No	Comments
Were Standard Precautions followed?			
Was equipment prepared correctly?			
Were the procedural steps properly followed?			
Was test control completed to verify results?			
Were contaminated items discarded correctly?			
Were test results accurately recorded?			

Evaluator:_______________________________ Date:_______________

Suggestions for improvement:____

CHAPTER 8 PERFORMING ROUTINE URINALYSIS

MATCHING

Match the terms in the right column with the definitions in the left column by writing the letters in the blanks.

Definitions	Terms
_____ 1. The color spectrum of urine.	a. Albumin
_____ 2. A systemic osmotic diuretic found in urine.	b. Bilirubin
_____ 3. Clouded or obscured.	c. Crenation
_____ 4. The excretion of urine exceeding 2000 mL in 24 hours.	d. Glycosuria
_____ 5. A water-soluble, heat-coagulable protein.	e. Polyuria
_____ 6. The formation of notches in red blood cells.	f. Urochrome
_____ 7. The orange-yellow pigment of bile formed by the breakdown of hemoglobin.	g. Supernatent
	h. Urea
_____ 8. The presence of sugar in urine.	i. Turbid
_____ 9. A measure that reflects a ratio of waste products to urinary fluid.	j. Specific gravity
_____10. The liquid portion of a centrifuged urine specimen.	

SHORT ANSWER

Answer the following questions:

11. Identify the condition that might be present when the urine specimen is:

Red or red-brown ______________________________

Clear pink or red ______________________________

Red or purple ______________________________

Dark brown or black ______________________________

Yellow-brown ______________________________

Dark yellow with white foam ______________________________

Green-brown ______________________________

12. Specific gravity is a convenient way of measuring the following:

____

13. List the qualitative tests performed in the chemical examination of urine and two conditions that may cause each test to be out of the average range.

____

____

____

____

14. How is a urine sample prepared for microscopic analysis?

____

____

____

____

15. Draw the following casts. Use colored pencils to illustrate.

hyaline	waxy	granular	erythrocyte

CRITICAL THINKING

Decide how you would handle the following situations, using the knowledge you have obtained in this chapter, combined with previously learned knowledge.

SITUATION # 1

This urine specimen is from a 27-year-old male who noted an increase in appetite and thirst over the past six months. He has only gained five pounds. He has complaints of increased urination, but says that he is not experiencing any pain when he urinates. A midstream cleancatch urine was obtained.

Macroscopic Urinalysis:		Microscopic Urinalysis:	
Color	Yellow	WBC/lpf	None
Appearance	Clear	RBC/lpf	1-2/lpf cells
Specific Gravity	1.008	Casts	None
pH	5.5	Other	None
Protein	Neg		
Glucose	4+		
Ketones	4+		
Bilirubin	Neg		
Blood	Neg		
Urobilinogen	Neg		
Nitrite	Neg		
Leukocyte Esterase	Neg		

1. What disease is suggested by these findings?

____

2. Will all sugars be detected by the reagent test strip for glucose? Why?

____

____

3. What is the significance of the positive test for ketones?

____

____

4. What are some complications of his disease that can affect the urinary system?

____

____

SITUATION #2

This 5-year-old boy usually drives his parents crazy by his hyperactivity, but for the past three weeks he has been very quiet and appears to have no energy. He has not been running a fever, but the mother has noted dark circles and puffiness around the eyes.

Macroscopic Urinalysis		**Microscopic Urinalysis**	
Color	Yellow	WBC/lpf	1-2/lpf
Appearance	Cloudy	RBC/lpf	None
Specific Gravity	1.020	Casts	None
pH	6.0	Other	Occasional oval fat bodies
Protein	4+		
Glucose	Neg		
Ketones	Neg		
Bilirubin	Neg		
Blood	Neg		
Urobilinogen	Neg		
Nitrite	Neg		
Leukocyte Esterase	Neg		

1. What abnormal finding is present?

   ____

2. What does this abnormal finding indicate?

   ____

3. What other test could be done on the urine to confirm the abnormal dipstick reading?

   ____

Procedure Evaluation Form

NAME:____

PROCEDURE:______________________________________

Technique	Yes	No	Comments
Were Standard Precautions followed?			
Was equipment prepared correctly?			
Were the procedural steps properly followed?			
Was test control completed to verify results?			
Were contaminated items discarded correctly?			
Were test results accurately recorded?			

Evaluator:____________________________ Date:_______________

Suggestions for improvement:____________________________

Procedure Evaluation Form

NAME:____

PROCEDURE:______________________________________

Technique	Yes	No	Comments
Were Standard Precautions followed?			
Was equipment prepared correctly?			
Were the procedural steps properly followed?			
Was test control completed to verify results?			
Were contaminated items discarded correctly?			
Were test results accurately recorded?			

Evaluator:____________________________ Date:_______________

Suggestions for improvement:____________________________

CHAPTER 9 SPECIALIZED URINE TESTS

MATCHING

Match the terms in the right column with the definitions in the left column by writing the letters in the blanks.

______ 1. Are mainly produced in the liver and bone marrow.

______ 2. Provides a more exact measure of urine concentration.

______ 3. A product of muscle energy metabolism.

______ 4. An abnormal increases in the body's hydrogen ion concentration resulting in a blood pH of < 7.4.

______ 5. An element which turns into ions that are able to conduct an electric current

______ 6. The clumping together of cells as a result of antibody and antigen interaction.

______ 7. The primary regulator of the body's ability to excrete or retain water.

______ 8. Functions as part of the buffer system of the body.

______ 9. A group of signs and symptoms resulting from a common cause or appearing in combinations.

______ 10. A test that determines the presence or absence of a substance.

a. Acidosis
b. Agglutination
c. Electrolyte
d. Qualitative test
e. Syndrome
f. Sodium
g. Potassium
h. Creatinine
i. Porphyrins
j. Osmolality

SHORT ANSWER

Answer the following questions:

11. Why is hCG a sign of early pregnancy?

____

____

12. Explain how and why agglutination indicates pregnancy.

____

____

____

13. Explain the reasons that urinary electrolyte measurements are quantitative tests.

____

14. What effect does the overproduction of porphyrins have on the body? What tests can be done to determine porphyrin levels?

15. List the reasons why urine is the most commonly used body fluid for drug screening.

CRITICAL THINKING

Decide how you would handle the following situations, using the knowledge you have obtained in this chapter, combined with previously learned knowledge.

SITUATION #1

A 29-year-old female comes to the office complaining of lower abdominal pain. She left her job as a nursing assistant (her first week on the job) because the pain was so bad. She says the pain began after she had fallen off a step stool while getting a bedpan off a top shelf. No one saw her fall, but she convinced her supervisor that she had an industrial accident and needed medical attention because of blood in her urine. To prove it, she brings in a urine specimen for analysis.

Macroscopic Urinalysis	
Color	Red
Appearance	Clear
Specific Gravity	1.015
pH	7.0
Protein	Neg
Glucose	Neg
Ketones	Neg
Bilirubin	Neg
Blood	Neg
Urobilinogen	Neg
Nitrite	Neg
Leukocyte Esterase	Neg

Microscopic Urinalysis	
WBC/lpf	Rare (<2/lpf)
RBC/lpf	None
Casts	Occasional hyaline casts
Other	Few squamous epithelial cells

1. How do you correlate the macroscopic and microscopic findings?

____

____

____

2. What do you think is going on here?

____

____

____

SITUATION #2

This 35-year-old male came to the doctor after spending a second sleepless night with excruciating lower abdominal pain. The pain seemed to come in waves and was unrelieved by aspirin, Acetaminophen, Ibuprofen, a six-pack of beer, or lying or standing in any position. He had not experienced any similar pain before.

Macroscopic Urinalysis		**Microscopic Urinalysis**	
Color	Dark Yellow	WBC/lpf	2-5/lpf
Appearance	Cloudy	RBC/lpf	>100/lpf
Specific Gravity	1.015	Casts	None
pH	6.0	Other	Occasional squamous epithelial cells
Protein	Neg		
Glucose	Neg		
Ketones	Neg		
Bilirubin	Neg		
Blood	3+		
Urobilinogen	Neg		
Nitrite	Neg		
Leukocyte Esterase	Neg		

1. What abnormal findings are present?

____

____

2. What diagnosis do you suspect?

____

____

3. What other lab studies might be done to confirm your suspected diagnosis?

____

____

Procedure Evaluation Form

NAME:____

PROCEDURE:____

Technique	Yes	No	Comments
Were Standard Precautions followed?			
Was equipment prepared correctly?			
Were the procedural steps properly followed?			
Was test control completed to verify results?			
Were contaminated items discarded correctly?			
Were test results accurately recorded?			

Evaluator:______________________________ Date:______________

Suggestions for improvement:______________________________

Procedure Evaluation Form

NAME:____

PROCEDURE:____

Technique	Yes	No	Comments
Were Standard Precautions followed?			
Was equipment prepared correctly?			
Were the procedural steps properly followed?			
Was test control completed to verify results?			
Were contaminated items discarded correctly?			
Were test results accurately recorded?			

Evaluator:______________________________ Date:______________

Suggestions for improvement:______________________________

UNIT III HEMATOLOGY

CHAPTER 10 ANATOMY AND PHYSIOLOGY OF THE BLOOD

MATCHING

Match the terms in the right column with the definitions in the left column by writing the letters in the blanks.

_____ 1. The most numerous of the leukocytes.	a. Phagocyte
_____ 2. Cells that are able to directly attack foreign matter and make antibodies.	b. Serum
	c. Agranulocytes
_____ 3. A protein produced by living cells.	d. Lymphocytes
_____ 4. Distributes oxygen throughout the body.	e. Enzyme
_____ 5. Transports various cell components throughout the body.	f. Hormone
_____ 6. A WBC that can ingest microorganisms and debris.	g. Erythrocytes
_____ 7. The end product of protein metabolism.	h. Urea
_____ 8. Mononuclear leukocytes that do not have dark-staining granules.	i. Granulocytes
_____ 9. A chemical substance secreted by an endocrine gland.	j. Plasma
_____10. Liquid portion of blood remaining after the clot formation process.	

SHORT ANSWERS

Answer the following questions.

11. List three types of granulocytes and the two types of agranulocytes and define the functions of these cells.

____

____

____

____

____

____

12. Identify five types of blood dyscrasias.

____

____

____

____

____

13. Describe the formation of platelets and explain their function.

____

____

____

14. Where does hematopoiesis occur in the body?

____

____

____

15. Identify each of the following cells and describe the major characteristics of its nucleus and cytoplasm.

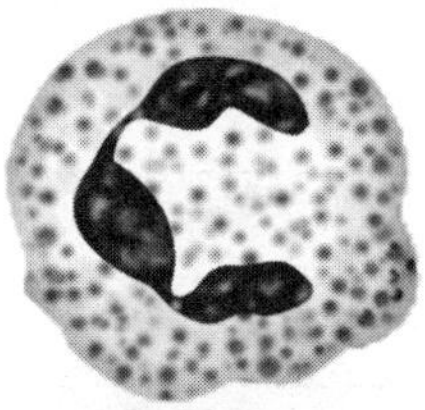

Name:______________________________

Nucleus:______________________________

Cytoplasm:______________________________

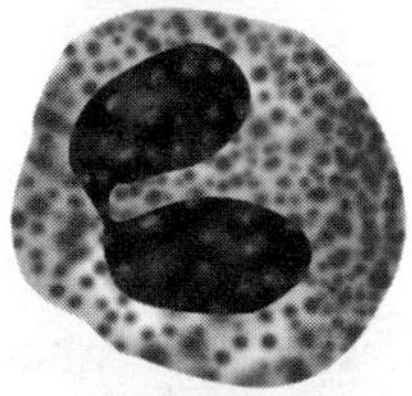

Name:______________________________

Nucleus:______________________________

Cytoplasm:______________________________

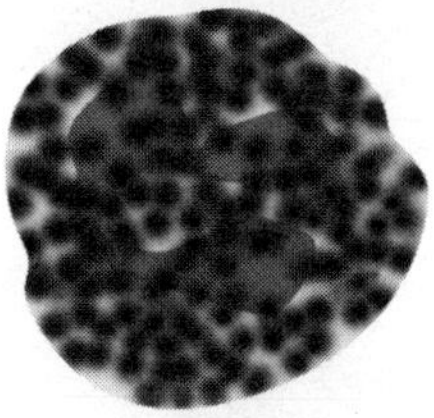

Name:______________________________

Nucleus:______________________________

Cytoplasm:______________________________

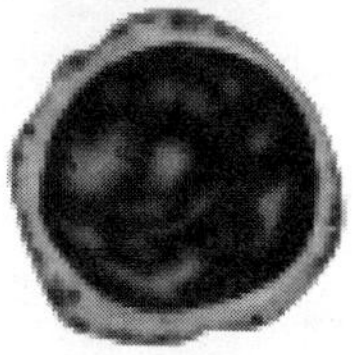

Name:______________________________

Nucleus:______________________________

Cytoplasm:______________________________

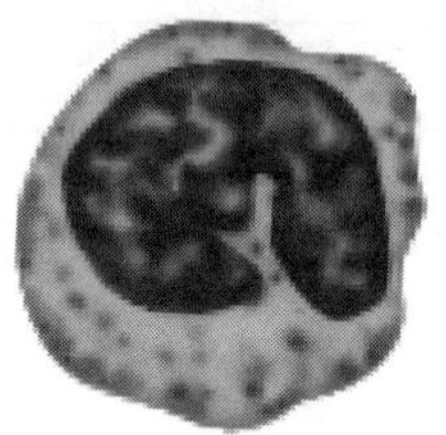

Name:____

Nucleus:______________________________________

Cytoplasm:_____________________________________

CRITICAL THINKING

Decide how you would handle the following situations, using the knowledge you have obtained in this chapter, combined with previously learned knowledge.

Situation #1

A complete blood count report comes back to the office from the laboratory and as you review the results, you notice that the RBC morphology is abnormal due to numerous reticulocytes counted. In addition, the differential white count shows the lymphocyte count to be 55%.

1. What are reticulocytes and when are they seen in a blood count?

____

____

____

2. What does an elevated lymphocyte count indicate?

____

____

3. If on a physical examination of this patient, enlarged lymph glands were seen, what might the diagnosis be?

____

Situation #2

Mr. D has been complaining of persistent headache and nasal congestion. His blood count shows a normal WBC but a large increase in eosinophils.

1. What is the patient most likely suffering from?

____

2. Are there other laboratory tests that could be ordered to substantiate this diagnosis? Name them.

____

____

____

Procedure Evaluation Form

NAME:____

PROCEDURE:____

Technique	Yes	No	Comments
Were StandardPprecautions followed?			
Was equipment prepared correctly?			
Were the procedural steps properly followed?			
Was test control completed to verify results?			
Were contaminated items discarded correctly?			
Were test results accurately recorded?			

Evaluator:______________________________ Date:______________

Suggestions for improvement:____

Procedure Evaluation Form

NAME:________________________

PROCEDURE:________________________

Technique	Yes	No	Comments
Were Standard Precautions followed?			
Was equipment prepared correctly?			
Were the procedural steps properly followed?			
Was test control completed to verify results?			
Were contaminated items discarded correctly?			
Were test results accurately recorded?			

Evaluator:____________________ Date:__________

Suggestions for improvement:____________________

Procedure Evaluation Form

NAME:________________________

PROCEDURE:________________________

Technique	Yes	No	Comments
Were Standard Precautions followed?			
Was equipment prepared correctly?			
Were the procedural steps properly followed?			
Was test control completed to verify results?			
Were contaminated items discarded correctly?			
Were test results accurately recorded?			

Evaluator:____________________ Date:__________

Suggestions for improvement:____________________

CHAPTER 11 BLOOD COLLECTION PROCEDURES

MATCHING

Match the terms in the right column with the definitions in the left column by writing the letters in the blanks.

_____ 1. The vein most often used for blood draw.	a. Cyanotic
_____ 2. Syringe mechanism that securely holds the needle in place.	b. Sclerosis
_____ 3. Most common blood collection system in use.	c. Heparin
_____ 4. Semiautomated device used for capillary puncture.	d. EDTA
_____ 5. A bluish discoloration of the skin and mucous membranes.	e. Syncope
_____ 6. Abnormal hardening of tissue.	f. Antecubital
_____ 7. A natural antithrombin factor that prevents intravascular clotting.	h. Autolet
_____ 8. An anticoagulant additive used when doing hematological studies.	i. Vacutainer
_____ 9. Fainting or temporary loss of consciousness.	j. Luer lock
_____10. In front of and at the bend of the elbow.	

SHORT ANSWER

Answer the following questions:

11. List four steps a laboratory assistant must know before attempting venipuncture.

____

____

____

____

12. When would you use a butterfly needle set?

____

____

____

13. What are two types of anticoagulant additives used for blood draw?

____

____

How are these two types color coded?

14. When would you select to draw the blood sample using a syringe?

Once you have the blood into the syringe, how do you prepare it for transfer to the laboratory?

15. It is extremely important that every blood sample be accurately labeled. What information should be included and when during the procedure do you label the specimen container?

CRITICAL THINKING

Decide how you would handle the following situations, using the knowledge you have obtained in this chapter, combined with previously learned knowledge.

Situation #1

Coach Jones comes in for his athletic physical and you are requested to obtain the samples for a CBC and a liver panel. He tells you that last night he was at a big alumni football party but made sure that he ate before midnight. He says he had one or two beers after midnight but was home before 2:00 AM and has had nothing to drink since then. He states that he is anxious to get this over with as he is starving. As you begin to draw the blood, he becomes very pale and slumps forward in the drawing chair.

1. What do you do immediately?

2. What measures could you have taken to minimize the risk of him fainting?

Situation #2

Jennifer, age 2, comes with her mother for a CBC with differential count. When she sees the tray of venipuncture supplies, she begins to cry and begs her mother to take her home.

1. What can you do to help Jennifer cope with this traumatizing situation?

____

____

2. What blood collection method would you choose to use? Why?

____

____

3. What precautions would you take for the child's safety?

____

____

Procedure Evaluation Form

NAME:____

PROCEDURE:____

Technique	**Yes**	**No**	**Comments**
Were Standard Precautions followed?			
Was equipment prepared correctly?			
Were the procedural steps properly followed?			
Was test control completed to verify results?			
Were contaminated items discarded correctly?			
Were test results accurately recorded?			

Evaluator:_______________________ Date:_______________

Suggestions for improvement:____

Procedure Evaluation Form

NAME:________________________________

PROCEDURE:________________________________

Technique	Yes	No	Comments
Were Standard Precautions followed?			
Was equipment prepared correctly?			
Were the procedural steps properly followed?			
Was test control completed to verify results?			
Were contaminated items discarded correctly?			
Were test results accurately recorded?			

Evaluator:____________________ Date:____________

Suggestions for improvement:____________________

Procedure Evaluation Form

NAME:________________________________

PROCEDURE:________________________________

Technique	Yes	No	Comments
Were Standard Precautions followed?			
Was equipment prepared correctly?			
Were the procedural steps properly followed?			
Was test control completed to verify results?			
Were contaminated items discarded correctly?			
Were test results accurately recorded?			

Evaluator:____________________ Date:____________

Suggestions for improvement:____________________

CHAPTER 12 HEMATOLOGIC TESTING PROCEDURES

MATCHING

Match the terms in the right column with the definitions in the left column by writing the letters in the blanks.

_____	1. Largest of the blood cell elements.	a. Bands
_____	2. Anemia in which the patient contains several different types of hemoglobin.	b. Thrombocytes
		c. Hemacytometer
_____	3. Immature forms of the neutrophil.	d. Thrombocytopenia
_____	4. Ingests bacteria and debris of cellular breakdown.	e. Leukopenia
_____	5. Increased number of platelets.	f. Erythrocytosis
_____	6. The most difficult of the cellular elements to count.	g. Monocytes
_____	7. Cell counting chamber with etched counting surface.	h. Thrombocytosis
_____	8. Abnormal increase in RBCs.	i. Leukocytes
_____	9. Decreased number of platelets.	j. Thalassemia
_____	10. Associated with viral infections or overexposure to therapeutic element.	

SHORT ANSWER

Answer the following questions:

11. The CBC is one of the most frequently performed laboratory tests. What tests does a CBC analysis contain?

____

____

____

12. List 5 types of anemia and the main causes of each.

____

____

____

____

____

13. Identify the three measurements of hemoglobin concentration.

____

____

____

14. List the three methods used to obtain a hemoglobin value.

____

____

____

15. Hematocrit and hemoglobin values that are out of the reference range indicate possible pathological conditions. Identify the possible disease that could cause each of these conditions.

High hemoglobin count: ______________________________

Low hemoglobin count: ______________________________

High hematocrit count: ______________________________

Low hematocrit count: ______________________________

A false high hemoglobin value: ______________________________

CRITICAL THINKING

Decide how you would handle the following situations, using the knowledge you have obtained in this chapter, combined with previously learned knowledge.

Situation #1

Find the MCV for a male patient with a hematocrit of 42% and an RBC of 5.0 million. What would the MCH and MCHC totals be for the same patient with a hemoglobin of 15?

____

____

Situation #2

Mark and Scott are working together in the laboratory. Mark has transferred a well-mixed, EDTA-anticoagulated blood specimen to a disposable Wintrobe tube. He places the tube up against the wall and sets the timer for one hour. Scott sees the tube standing against the wall and places it in a sed rack. When the hour is up, Mark looks for the tube but can't locate it. Scott tells him he placed it in the sed rack.

Mark is furious and says that the test is no longer valid due to the fact that the tube was moved during the settling period. Scott says that if he hadn't put the tube into the rack, it would have be invalid and that this way the test is accurate. Who is right? Justify your answer.

____

____

____

Procedure Evaluation Form

NAME:____

PROCEDURE:____

Technique	Yes	No	Comments
Were Standard Precautions followed?			
Was equipment prepared correctly?			
Were the procedural steps properly followed?			
Was test control completed to verify results?			
Were contaminated items discarded correctly?			
Were test results accurately recorded?			

Evaluator:______________________ Date:______________

Suggestions for improvement:____

Procedure Evaluation Form

NAME:____

PROCEDURE:____

Technique	Yes	No	Comments
Were Standard Precautions followed?			
Was equipment prepared correctly?			
Were the procedural steps properly followed?			
Was test control completed to verify results?			
Were contaminated items discarded correctly?			
Were test results accurately recorded?			

Evaluator:______________________ Date:______________

Suggestions for improvement:____

CHAPTER 13 COAGULATION TESTING

MATCHING

Match the terms in the right column with the definitions in the left column by writing the letters in the blanks.

______	1. An inflammation and congestion of a vessel.	a. Edema
______	2. Clustering or clumping of blood cells.	b. Embolus
______	3. Formation of plaque on the inside walls of arteries.	c. ADP
______	4. Foreign object circulating in the blood stream.	d. Coagulation
______	5. A congenital defect characterized by dwarfing.	e. Hemostasis
______	6. Conversion of liquid blood into semi-solid gel.	f. Artherosclerosis
______	7. An instrument used to perform coagulation tests.	g. Vasculitis
______	8. Excessive fluid accumulation in tissue.	h. Aggregation
______	9. A product of the hydrolysis of adenosine triphosphate.	i. Diastema
______	10. The body's mechanism for terminating bleeding.	j. Fibrometer

SHORT ANSWER

Answer the following questions:

11. The conversion of fibrinogen to fibrin is the end result of a common pathway, and both intrinsic and extrinsic pathways must work together to activate the common pathway. Explain the steps in this conversion.

____

____

____

____

12. Female hemophiliacs are extremely rare. Why?

____

____

13. The normal clotting time is ____________________. When the clotting time is prolonged, the likely cause is:

____

14. Identify the three most commonly used coagulation tests and indicate the reference range for each.

_______________ _______________ _______________

Range:_______________ Range:_______________ Range:_______________

15. Define bleeding time.

____

16. Name the two bleeding time tests discussed in your text and indicate the reference range for each.

_______________ _______________

Range:_______________ Range:_______________

17. Explain how coagulation studies are done manually.

____

____

18. Describe the relationship between heparin and Coumadin and how these two drugs are monitored using coagulation studies.

____

____

____

CRITICAL THINKING

Decide how you would handle the following situations, using the knowledge you have obtained in this chapter, combined with previously learned knowledge.

Situation #1

A patient comes in for his preoperative blood studies for open heart surgery. You prepare the patient and make conversation with him as you prepare for the draws. One of the tests ordered is a bleeding time test. The patient tells you that he is worried about the arthritic condition in his knees because he will be unable to actively walk during his immediate recovery period. He tells you that he is still taking his Ibuprofen 800 mg daily and plans to take it with him to the hospital because his arthritis doctor told him not to miss a day.

1. Does this information relate to the tests ordered? Explain.

____

____

2. What would be your choice of action?

____

____

Situation #2

This has been a real hectic day in the laboratory and the day is almost over. As you are checking all of the work orders, you discover that you were suppose to do a protime on Mrs. Bee and fax the results to the physician before 5:00 PM today. It is now 4:00 PM, your duty day is ending, and Mrs. Bee's blood is still in the refrigerator. Knowing that the blood must be room temperature before the test can be done, you must make some definite decisions regarding this forgotten test. What would you do?

____

____

____

____

____

Procedure Evaluation Form

NAME:____

PROCEDURE:____

Technique	**Yes**	**No**	**Comments**
Were Standard Precautions followed?			
Was equipment prepared correctly?			
Were the procedural steps properly followed?			
Was test control completed to verify results?			
Were contaminated items discarded correctly?			
Were test results accurately recorded?			

Evaluator:__________________________________ Date:__________________

Suggestions for improvement:____

Procedure Evaluation Form

NAME:______________________________

PROCEDURE:______________________________

Technique	Yes	No	Comments
Were Standard Precautions followed?			
Was equipment prepared correctly?			
Were the procedural steps properly followed?			
Was test control completed to verify results?			
Were contaminated items discarded correctly?			
Were test results accurately recorded?			

Evaluator:____________________ Date:________________

Suggestions for improvement:____________________

Procedure Evaluation Form

NAME:______________________________

PROCEDURE:______________________________

Technique	Yes	No	Comments
Were Standard Precautions followed?			
Was equipment prepared correctly?			
Were the procedural steps properly followed?			
Was test control completed to verify results?			
Were contaminated items discarded correctly?			
Were test results accurately recorded?			

Evaluator:____________________ Date:________________

Suggestions for improvement:____________________

UNIT IV BLOOD CHEMISTRY

CHAPTER 14 INTRODUCTION TO CLINICAL CHEMISTRY

MATCHING

Match the terms in the right column with the definitions in the left column by writing the letters in the blanks.

______ 1. Reversal of the normal specimen position.		a. Hemolysis
______ 2. Nonprotein, insoluble, iron protoporphyrin.		b. Green-top
______ 3. A sample that is representative of the whole.		c. Icterus
______ 4. Neither translucent nor transparent.		d. Hyperlipidemia
______ 5. Cloudy, not clear.		e. Red-top
______ 6. Will cause plasma to be pink or red.		f. Aliquot
______ 7. Vacutainer coded for uncoagulated blood.		g. Heme
______ 8. Caused by high levels of bilirubin.		h. Turbid
______ 9. Will cause plasma to be deep yellow or orange.		i. Opaque
______10. Vacutainer coded for coagulated blood.		j. Inversion

SHORT ANSWER

Answer the following questions:

11. List the materials and equipment necessary for a mid-stream urine specimen collection.

____

____

____

12. Identify the reference range for the following:

a. Serum glucose for a 10-year-old ______________________________

b. Uric acid for a 30-year-old ______________________________

c. Serum potassium for a 60-year-old ______________________________

d. BUN for a 6-month-old ______________________________

e. Uric acid for a 40-year-old ______________________________

13. The ideal refrigerator temperature for specimen storage is ______________________

14. The ideal freezer temperature for specimen storage is ______________________

15. The laboratory centrifuge must be capable of speeds of ______________________

16. The reason stat requests involve using plasma over serum is______________________

17. Why is it necessary to use a syringe, not a Vacutainer, when obtaining an arterial blood collection?

____

____

18. All urine specimens should be handled with caution. Why?

____

____

19. Why have reference ranges been established for each test? What does it mean when results are not in this range?

____

____

20. A 24-hour urine test for porphyrin assay has been ordered. How would you prepare the container and what instructions would you give the patient?

____

____

____

____

CRITICAL THINKING

Decide how you would handle the following situations, using the knowledge you have obtained in this chapter, combined with previously learned knowledge.

Situation #1

Within the area that you live, what are the regulations and protocols regarding eligibility to perform arterial specimen collection? (You will find this information in the protocols of reference laboratories.)

____

____

Situation #2

Mrs. Fargo comes to the laboratory, during her lunch hour, with a request for a chemistry panel. She states that she had only a salad for lunch. What would your draw consist of? How many milliliters and what tube-top colors would you use? After the draw, you spin the blood and the plasma has a turbid appearance. Is this abnormal or significant? What might be the reason?

Procedure Evaluation Form

NAME:____________________

PROCEDURE:____________________

Technique	Yes	No	Comments
Were Standard Precautions followed?			
Was equipment prepared correctly?			
Were the procedural steps properly followed?			
Was test control completed to verify results?			
Were contaminated items discarded correctly?			
Were test results accurately recorded?			

Evaluator:____________________ Date:__________

Suggestions for improvement:____________________

CHAPTER 15 BASIC CHEMISTRY LABORATORY INSTRUMENTATION

MATCHING

Match the terms in the right column with the definitions in the left column by writing the letters in the blanks.

_____ 1. Test method in which an enzyme is added and peak of reaction is measured.

_____ 2. To measure a measurable amount of mass.

_____ 3. Separating matter by slowly running water over it.

_____ 4. Convex surface in a tube or pipette.

_____ 5. Test method in which serum is added to certain enzymes which frees an analyte for analysis of end color.

_____ 6. Pipette allowed to drain by gravity; do not require rinsing.

_____ 7. An indication of the reproducibility of a measurement.

_____ 8. Test in which a darker reaction color indicates more of the absorbing substance is present.

_____ 9. Pipette that must be rinsed.

_____10. Capable of emitting light or heat rays.

a. Enzymatic method

b. Meniscus

c. TD

d. TC

e. Kinetic method

f. Colorimetric

g. Radiant

h. Leaching

i. Reliability

j. Quantitate

SHORT ANSWER

Answer the following questions.

11. List five methods of lab testing.

____

____

____

____

____

12. Describe the three types of pipettes and the uses for each.

____

____

____

13. Express the following in complete terms using the International System of Nomenclature

a. Bun 10 mg/dL ____________________

b. Serum chloride 103 mEq/L ____________________

c. Uric acid 5.7 mg/dL ____________________

14. Which method of testing would be most appropriated for checking the volume of sodium in a sample. Explain the process.

____

____

____

15. Explain the differences between volumetric and graduated pipettes.

____

____

____

CRITICAL THINKING

Decide how you would handle the following situations, using the knowledge you have obtained in this chapter, combined with previously learned knowledge.

Situation #1

On the laboratory test result form, indicate the nomenclature measurement for each of the test results listed.

TEST	RESULTS	UNITS
	------CHEMISTRY PANEL------	
Glucose	80	______
Potassium	4.8	______
Chloride	100	______
Uric acid	5.7	______
Alkaline Phos	82	______
Albumin	5.1	______
Iron	126	______
Cholesterol	257	______

1. Are all the tests within reference range?

____

ituation #2

ou need 500 mL of a 5% solution of hydrochloric acid (HCL) for testing analysis. On hand is HCL 20% olution. How could is be prepared?

rocedure Evaluation Form

AME:______________________________

ROCEDURE:______________________________

echnique	Yes	No	Comments
/ere Standard Precautions followed?			
/as equipment prepared correctly?			
/ere the procedural steps properly followed?			
/as test control completed to verify results?			
/ere contaminated items discarded correctly?			
/ere test results accurately recorded?			

valuator:____________________ Date:__________

uggestions for improvement:____________________

CHAPTER 16 ROUTINE CLINICAL CHEMISTRY PROCEDURES

MATCHING

Match the terms in the right column with the definitions in the left column by writing the letters in the blanks.

_____ 1. Positively charged ions.	a. Fast
_____ 2. Negatively charged ions.	b. Urea
_____ 3. Abstinence from food or nourishment.	c. Gout
_____ 4. Largest constituent routinely measured.	d. Dehydration
_____ 5. Chief nitrogenous end product of protein metabolism.	e. Ketoacidosis
_____ 6. Most frequent urine test ordered in the lab.	f. Protein
_____ 7. Results from undue loss of water from the body.	g. Cations
_____ 8. Most frequent panel ordered in lab.	h. Renal
_____ 9. Accumulation of fatty acids.	i. Glucose
_____10. A hereditary disorder caused by excessive uric acid in the blood.	j. Anions

SHORT ANSWER

Answer the following questions:

11. List four liver enzyme tests and describe the testing procedure used for each one.

____

____

____

____

12. Explain how the measurement of the enzymes LDH and CPK is used to detect myocardial infarction.

____

____

____

____

CRITICAL THINKING

Decide how you would handle the following situations, using the knowledge you have obtained in this chapter, combined with previously learned knowledge.

Situation #1

List a possible diagnosis for the following test results:

1. Blood cholesterol level of 245 mg/dL in a 53-year-old male ______________________
2. Uric acid of 8.7 mg/dL in a 48-year-old-male ______________________
3. Serum glucose of 120 mg/dL in an 11-year-old child______________________
4. Serum sodium of 215 mEq/L in a 41-year-old female______________________
5. LDH of 295 mU/mL in a 17-year-old male______________________

Situation #2

1. A 56-year-old female has a history of heart palpitations and angina. The cardiac chemistry panel indicates an LDL level of 240 mg/dL and an HDL of 92 mg/dL. Determine the cardiac risk factor following this formula: LDL ÷ HDL = RF(risk factor)

2. A 56-year-old male has a similar history of heart palpitations with angina. The cardiac chemistry panel indicates that his LDL level is 230 mg/dL and his HDL is 75 mg/dL. Determine his cardiac risk factor. LDL ÷ HDL = RF(risk factor)

3. The higher the RF the greater the risk of heart attack. Which patient is at greater risk? What could be the reason?

____

____

Procedure Evaluation Form

NAME:________________________________

PROCEDURE:________________________________

Technique	Yes	No	Comments
Were Standard Precautions followed?			
Was equipment prepared correctly?			
Were the procedural steps properly followed?			
Was test control completed to verify results?			
Were contaminated items discarded correctly?			
Were test results accurately recorded?			

Evaluator:________________________ Date:____________

Suggestions for improvement:________________________

Procedure Evaluation Form

NAME:________________________________

PROCEDURE:________________________________

Technique	Yes	No	Comments
Were Standard Precautions followed?			
Was equipment prepared correctly?			
Were the procedural steps properly followed?			
Was test control completed to verify results?			
Were contaminated items discarded correctly?			
Were test results accurately recorded?			

Evaluator:________________________ Date:____________

Suggestions for improvement:________________________

Procedure Evaluation Form

NAME:____

PROCEDURE:____________________________________

Technique	Yes	No	Comments
Were Standard Precautions followed?			
Was equipment prepared correctly?			
Were the procedural steps properly followed?			
Was test control completed to verify results?			
Were contaminated items discarded correctly?			
Were test results accurately recorded?			

Evaluator:______________________________ Date:________________

Suggestions for improvement:______________________________

Procedure Evaluation Form

NAME:____

PROCEDURE:____________________________________

Technique	Yes	No	Comments
Were Standard Precautions followed?			
Was equipment prepared correctly?			
Were the procedural steps properly followed?			
Was test control completed to verify results?			
Were contaminated items discarded correctly?			
Were test results accurately recorded?			

Evaluator:______________________________ Date:________________

Suggestions for improvement:______________________________

CHAPTER 17 TOXICOLOGY

MATCHING

Match the terms in the right column with the definitions in the left column by writing the letters in the blanks.

_____ 1. A precise measurement that determines the amount of substance present or absent.	a. Methadone
	b. Quantitative
_____ 2. Synthetic narcotic used to prevent withdrawal symptoms.	c. Qualitative
_____ 3. Tetrahydrocannabinol is the main active ingredient.	d. Methanol
_____ 4. Synthetic drug used as a substitute for ephedrine	e. Methamphetamine
_____ 5. An ingredient in antifreeze.	f. Suppressant
_____ 6. Method of choice for forensic blood alcohol testing.	g. Decongestant
_____ 7. A substance capable of dissolving another material.	h. Solvent
_____ 8. An agent that stops secretion and excretion.	i. Gas chromatography
_____ 9. A precise physical measurement of energy or mass.	j. Cannabis
_____10. An agent that reduces swelling.	

SHORT ANSWER

Answer the following questions:

11. What specifics are necessary to label a specimen positive for a drug?

____

____

12. List four common immunoassays.

____

____

____

____

13. The cholinesterase test is commonly performed in clinical laboratories to detect the following:

____

____

14. Name four poisonous metals. Are any of these toxic for very young children?

____

____

15. The most widely used and abused drug is ______________________________.

16. A major component in perfumes and aftershaves is ______________________.

17. Chronic use of methamphetamine can induce _____________________________.

18. The anesthetic of choice for types of oropharyngeal surgery is ______________.

19. Morphine, codeine, and heroin, are all derivatives of ______________________.

20. Medical uses of marijuana have included the following:

____

____

____

____

CRITICAL THINKING

Decide how you would handle the following situations, using the knowledge you have obtained in this chapter, combined with previously learned knowledge.

Situation #1

Mr. M has a positive urine result for methamphetamine. Mrs. S has a positive urine result for morphine. Mr. O has a positive urine result for alcohol. All three were found to be false positives. Which patient would be most likely followed up with more studies? Why?

____

____

Situation #2

The local police officer brings in a female who is suspected of being under the influence of drugs and alcohol. You are given the necessary paperwork and take her back into the bathroom to collect a urine sample. The woman is menstruating. What do you do?

____

____

Procedure Evaluation Form

NAME:____________________________

PROCEDURE:____________________________

Technique	Yes	No	Comments
Were Standard Precautions followed?			
Was equipment prepared correctly?			
Were the procedural steps properly followed?			
Was test control completed to verify results?			
Were contaminated items discarded correctly?			
Were test results accurately recorded?			

Evaluator:____________________________ Date:______________

Suggestions for improvement:____________________________

Procedure Evaluation Form

NAME:____________________________

PROCEDURE:____________________________

Technique	Yes	No	Comments
Were Standard Precautions followed?			
Was equipment prepared correctly?			
Were the procedural steps properly followed?			
Was test control completed to verify results?			
Were contaminated items discarded correctly?			
Were test results accurately recorded?			

Evaluator:____________________________ Date:______________

Suggestions for improvement:____________________________

CHAPTER 18 THERAPEUTIC DRUG MONITORING

MATCHING

Match the terms in the right column with the definitions in the left column by writing the letters in the blanks.

_____ 1. Drug evaluated by steady-state peak concentration.	a. TDM
_____ 2. Drug whose dosage is gauged by a therapeutic window.	b. Pharmacokinetics
_____ 3. Responds to steady-state dosing.	c. Gentamycin
_____ 4. The mechanism of the drug's action in the body.	d. Metabolism
_____ 5. Fate of drug in the kidney.	e. Half-life
_____ 6. The level at which a drug becomes poisonous in the body.	f. Diazepam
_____ 7. The quantitative study of drug disposition in the body.	g. Liberation
_____ 8. Release of drug from its dosage.	h. Elimination
_____ 9. The time it takes to eliminate 50% of a drug.	i. Toxicity
_____10. Breakdown of drug in the liver.	j. Bacterial antibiotics

SHORT ANSWER

Answer the following questions:

11. List the guidelines for drug monitoring.

____

____

____

____

12. Describe the different dosing regiments and name a drug classified for each regiment.

____

____

____

____.

13. If Mr. G. has just begun digoxin therapy, what would be his optimal sampling time? Explain.

____

____

____

14. Choose a family member that you know takes a considerable amount of medications. Make a list of the medications that this person uses everyday and on a frequent basis. Compare this list with the half-life list in your text. How many of these drugs appear on the list? Has this person ever been tested for drug compatibility or dosing regime?

____

____

____

____

15. You are to draw a peak level on Ms. T. What equipment and supplies will you need for this draw?

____

____

____

____

CRITICAL THINKING

Decide how you would handle the following situations, using the knowledge you have obtained in this chapter, combined with previously learned knowledge.

Situation #1

Mrs. D is on Valium and the physician wants to know the blood level of the drug. A peak and trough sampling is ordered. She takes Valium by intramuscular injection every six hours, at 7:00 and at 1:00 both AM and PM. When would you do the draws? What equipment would you need? How would you handle the sample after the draw? Would you have Mrs. D stay at the lab until you complete both draws? Why?

____

____

____

____

____

____

Situation #2

You are asked to post the Peak and Trough test results to the patient's medical records. Decide which of the following you would put on the physician's desk for review and if any of these results need to be shown to him STAT.

	Drug:	Test Results:	Action Taken
Mr. J. B.	Gentamycin (garamycin)	6.4 ug/mL	______________
Ms. S.B.	Amytal (amobarital sodium)	10 ug/mL	______________
Mrs. L.L.	Tofranil (imipramine hydrochloride)	350 ng/mL	______________
Mr. A.B.	Quinaglute (quinidine sulfate)	0.9 ug/mL	______________

Procedure Evaluation Form

NAME:______________________________

PROCEDURE:______________________________

Technique	Yes	No	Comments
Were Standard Precautions followed?			
Was equipment prepared correctly?			
Were the procedural steps properly followed?			
Was test control completed to verify results?			
Were contaminated items discarded correctly?			
Were test results accurately recorded?			

Evaluator:______________________________ Date:______________

Suggestions for improvement:______________________________

CHAPTER 19 SPECIALIZED TESTING

MATCHING

Match the terms in the right column with the definitions in the left column by writing the letters in the blanks.

Definitions	Terms
______ 1. Amount of oxygen bound to hemoglobin and available for transport in the blood.	a. PO_2
______ 2. A hormone secreted by the posterior lobe of the pituitary.	b. SO_2
______ 3. Amount of oxygen dissolved in plasma that reflects the status of alveolar gas exchange with inspired air.	c. Osmolality
______ 4. Immobility or stiffening of a joint.	d. HLA
______ 5. A fluorescent antinuclear antibody study.	e. PSA
______ 6. Inflammation of the vertebrae.	f. Electrophoresis
______ 7. Technique used to identify a substance based on its migration in an electric field.	g. Ankylosing
______ 8. Test used to diagnose prostate cancer.	h. Spondylitis
______ 9. Measure of the number of dissolved particles in a solution.	i. ADH
______10. Test used to diagnose multiple sclerosis.	j. FANA

SHORT ANSWER

Answer the following questions:

11. How are fluorescent antibody studies used to detect lupus?

____

____

____

12 Explain the procedure for RIA analysis.

____

____

____

13. Osmolality is a measure of____.

It is closely associated with ______________________________

and ______________________________.

14. List the steps in the development of paternity testing.

____

____

____

15. How does the PSA test differ from the PAP test for prostate-specific antigen?

____

____

____

CRITICAL THINKING

Decide how you would handle the following situations, using the knowledge you have obtained in this chapter, combined with previously learned knowledge.

Situation #1

Two samples marked A and B were tested using the HLA system. The two samples were found to have perfect tissue compatibility. What determination can be made about the two people who submitted the samples A and B?

____

____

____

Situation #2

The Results of Mr. A.F.'s arterial blood gas analysis is:

Test	Results	Reference range	Evaluation
pH	7.25	__________	__________
O_2 Content	10 vol %	__________	__________
PO_2	81 torr	__________	__________
SO_2	89% of capacity	__________	__________
CO_2	45 nmol/L	__________	__________
Pco_2	40 mm Hg	__________	__________
HCO_3	30 mEq/L	__________	__________
Base excess	2.5 mEq/L	__________	__________
Base deficit	3.3 mEq/L	__________	__________

1. Fill in the reference values and in the evaluation column, indicate whether it was within the reference range, excess, or deficient.
2. Looking at the results of this analysis, do you feel that the test results are justified or do you feel the test needs to be rerun? Why?

____

____

____

Procedure Evaluation Form

NAME:______________________________

PROCEDURE:______________________________

Technique	Yes	No	Comments
Were Standard Precautions followed?			
Was equipment prepared correctly?			
Were the procedural steps properly followed?			
Was test control completed to verify results?			
Were contaminated items discarded correctly?			
Were test results accurately recorded?			

Evaluator:____________________ Date:__________

Suggestions for improvement:____________________

Procedure Evaluation Form

NAME:______________________________

PROCEDURE:______________________________

Technique	Yes	No	Comments
Were Standard Precautions followed?			
Was equipment prepared correctly?			
Were the procedural steps properly followed?			
Was test control completed to verify results?			
Were contaminated items discarded correctly?			
Were test results accurately recorded?			

Evaluator:____________________ Date:__________

Suggestions for improvement:____________________

UNIT V SEROLOGY AND IMMUNOHEMATOLOGY

CHAPTER 20 INTRODUCTION TO SEROLOGY AND IMMUNOHEMATOLOGY

MATCHING

Match the terms in the right column with the definitions in the left column by writing the letters in the blanks

_____ 1. Ability of a test to identify the condition or disease being tested.

_____ 2. An antibody-producing cell.

_____ 3. Antibodies developed after a previous infection.

_____ 4. Proteins that stimulate T-cell lymphocytes.

_____ 5. Lymphocytes that destroy antigens.

_____ 6. Lymphocytes that secrete antigens.

_____ 7. The substance quantity required to react to another substance.

_____ 8. Protests the body against infections by vaccination.

_____ 9. Ability of a test to distinguish between the specific antibody or antigen being tested from all the others being tested.

_____10. Proteins that can stimulate macrophages to eat bacteria.

a. T-cells
b. Interferon
c. Sensitivity
d. B-cells
e. Active immunity
f. Interleukins
g. Specificity
h. Titer
i. Passive immunity
j. Plasma cell

SHORT ANSWER

Answer the following questions:

11. Compare and contrast the location and function of the different types of immunity.

____

____

____

____

12. Identify the two major types of lymphocytes. How are the functions of each alike and how are they different?

____

____

____

13. If you are exposed to hepatitis and require an immunoglobulin injection, which one would you receive? Why?

____

____

____

____

14. Why is the blood bank a specialized area within immunology?

____

____

____

____

15. Describe the functions of the macrophage cell.

____

____

____

____

CRITICAL THINKING

Decide how you would handle the following situations, using the knowledge you have obtained in this chapter, combined with previously learned knowledge.

Situation #1

Ms. M., a health care worker, was found to be positive for hepatitis B antibodies. Her father had hepatitis B before she was born. What type of immune response would be most appropriate in Ms. M.'s case? Justify your answer.

____

____

____

____

Situation #2

John is 10 years old and has an allergy to bee stings. His family has had him tested, and he is to receive allergy shots to desensitize him. In these shots, he will be given small amounts of the offending antigen and the concentration will be gradually increased. Explain what this antigen will do to his immune system to eliminate his allergy.

____

____

____

____

Procedure Evaluation Form

NAME:____

PROCEDURE:____

Technique	Yes	No	Comments
Were Standard Precautions followed?			
Was equipment prepared correctly?			
Were the procedural steps properly followed?			
Was test control completed to verify results?			
Were contaminated items discarded correctly?			
Were test results accurately recorded?			

Evaluator:______________________________ Date:______________

Suggestions for improvement:____

CHAPTER 21 SEROLOGIC TESTING AND PROCEDURES

MATCHING

Match the terms in the right column with the definitions in the left column by writing the letters in the blanks.

_____ 1. Biological reaction that occurs in a living body.

_____ 2. Light generated as a result of a chemical reaction.

_____ 3. Organic compound with luminescent qualities.

_____ 4. Biological reaction that occurs in an artificial environment.

_____ 5. Reaction found in nature between an enzyme and an oxygen -producing cold light.

_____ 6. Poisonous substances secreted externally.

_____ 7. An antibody that reacts with antigens other than the one it is expected to react with.

_____ 8. Clumping of blood cells caused by an antigen/antibody reaction.

_____ 9. Hormone produced in the chorionic villi of the placenta.

_____10. A chronic destructive and deforming systemic collagen disease.

a. Exotoxins
b. In vitro
c. Heterophil
d. In vivo
e. Agglutination
f. Bioluminescence
g. hCG
h. Chemiluminescence
i. Rheumatoid arthritis
j. Luminal

SHORT ANSWER

Answer the following questions:

11. List four serological testing methods and the infections they identify.

Testing Method	Commonly Used to Identify
________________	________________________________
________________	________________________________
________________	________________________________
________________	________________________________

12. What does a false-positive test result indicate?

____

13. How are immune reactions measured quantitatively?

____

____

14. How and why do you neutralize an antigen?

____

____

CRITICAL THINKING

Decide how you would handle the following situations, using the knowledge you have obtained in this chapter, combined with previously learned knowledge.

Situation # 1

Mrs. O presents with complaints of fatigue, malaise, loss of appetite, fever, and joint pain. She is exhibiting early symptoms of what disease? List the tests that might be used to confirm her condition.

____

____

____

Situation #2

Conduct a quality control check in immunology testing in a POL. What methods were employed? Are the same standards followed in the laboratory as at school? If there is a difference, explain the rationale for the differences.

____

____

____

____

Procedure Evaluation Form

NAME:____

PROCEDURE:____

Technique	**Yes**	**No**	**Comments**
Were Standard Precautions followed?			
Was equipment prepared correctly?			
Were the procedural steps properly followed?			
Was test control completed to verify results?			
Were contaminated items discarded correctly?			
Were test results accurately recorded?			

Evaluator:____________________________ Date:________________

Suggestions for improvement:____

Procedure Evaluation Form

NAME:____

PROCEDURE:____

Technique	**Yes**	**No**	**Comments**
Were Standard Precautions followed?			
Was equipment prepared correctly?			
Were the procedural steps properly followed?			
Was test control completed to verify results?			
Were contaminated items discarded correctly?			
Were test results accurately recorded?			

Evaluator:____________________________ Date:________________

Suggestions for improvement:____

CHAPTER 22 IMMUNOHEMATOLOGIC TESTING AND PROCEDURES

MATCHING

Match the terms in the right column with the definitions in the left column by writing the letters in the blanks.

_____ 1. Rh system antigens.

_____ 2. Self-donated blood for later transfusion.

_____ 3. Blood type containing neither anti-A nor anti-B antibodies.

_____ 4. Indicates blood incompatibility.

_____ 5. Rh incompatibility between mother and first newborn may result in this disease in succeeding children.

_____ 6. Pertains to the legal aspects of a given test or procedure.

_____ 7. Refer to the presence or absence of RBC antigen D.

_____ 8. Blood type containing both anti-A and anti-B antibodies.

_____ 9. Discovered three groups of human bloods.

_____10. Hemolytic anemia resulting from fetal-maternal blood group incompatibility.

a. Karl Landsteiner

b. Type AB

c. Rh

d. Autologous

e. HDN

f. Hemolytic

g. D, C, c, E, e

h. Type O

i. Agglutination

j. Forensic

SHORT ANSWER

Answer the following questions:

11. What are the major clinical reasons for performing blood bank tests?

____

____

____

12. Identify the major human blood groups.

______________________________ ______________________________

______________________________ ______________________________

13. List the steps for Rh type determination.

____

____

____

14. Antibodies of the ABO system are naturally occurring. Antibodies of the Rh system are not. List the ways a person might develop Rh antibodies.

____

____

____

15. HDN can cause severe problems in the newborn. What are two possible results of this disease?

____

____

16. A woman who is Rh negative will be given an injection of this prenatally (before the baby is born), after an Rh-positive baby is born, or after an abortion, to prevent development of Rh antibodies that cause HDN. What is in the injection?

____

17. What are the symptoms of a transfusion reaction?

____

18. What tests are performed when doing crossmatch testing?

____

CRITICAL THINKING

Decide how you would handle the following situations, using the knowledge you have obtained in this chapter, combined with previously learned knowledge.

Situation #1

Mr. Q requires a donation of blood for emergency hip surgery. He is Type AB. There are three pints of blood available, one Type A, one Type B, and one Type O. Which blood can be donated and why?

____

____

____

Situation #2

Mary is scheduled for surgery in several weeks. She has come to the office with several of her family members and two friends. Mary wants her blood type and the blood type of her family and friends so that they may donate blood for her. Mary will also be giving a unit of her own blood for transfusion if needed. One of Mary's friends proudly announces that she has type O blood. She declares that type O blood, given as packed cells, is known as the universal donor and that Mary surely will be able to receive her blood. Mary's blood is tested and she is found to be A positive. All of the blood Mary will receive will ne in the form of packed red blood cells. This means the plasma that contains the antibodies has been removed and Mary will be transfused with only the red blood cells.

1. What is the name for the transfusion that involves Mary receiving her own blood?

 ____

2. What blood groups must Mary's friends and family be in order for her to receive their blood in the form of packed red blood cells?

 ____

3. What antigens are on the cells of Mary's friend that make her a universal donor? Explain.

 ____

 ____

4. What type of antibodies does Mary's blood have?

 ____

 ____

Situation #3

The technologist from the local hospital has faxed over a copy of a blood grouping and typing on one of your patients. Unfortunately the technologist forgot to write down his interpretation of the reactions. Although you realize that the results must be interpreted by the doctor or lab technologist, you would like to try out your new found knowledge of blood banking. The "ANTI-" section means you take antisera A and antisera B and place these into separate test tubes , and the patient's cells are then added to each test tube to determine the blood group. Anti D and a control (CTL) were used to determine the Rh type. A and B cells were tested with the patient's serum. The tubes were spun, checked for hemolysis or agglutination, and the results written down as follows:

PROCEDURE (CIRCLE)								ANTIBODY SCREEN LOT # ________				
ABO/RH			CRDTYPE									
ANTI-					CELLS	INT		CELL	37	IGG	CC	INT
A	B	D	CTL	DU	A1	B	ABO/ RH	I				
								II				
3+	0	2+	0		0	3+		________				
								III				
								________				

1. What blood group is the patient?

____

2. What Rh type is the patient?

____

3. If you were to look at the tube that had the three plus reaction, describe the clumping you would see.

____

4. The cells that were tested against the B cells show agglutination. What antibody is present in the serum to cause this?

____

Procedure Evaluation Form

NAME:____

PROCEDURE:____

Technique	Yes	No	Comments
Were Standard Precautions followed?			
Was equipment prepared correctly?			
Were the procedural steps properly followed?			
Was test control completed to verify results?			
Were contaminated items discarded correctly?			
Were test results accurately recorded?			

Evaluator:____________________________ Date:______________

Suggestions for improvement:____________________________

Procedure Evaluation Form

NAME:____

PROCEDURE:____

Technique	Yes	No	Comments
Were Standard Precautions followed?			
Was equipment prepared correctly?			
Were the procedural steps properly followed?			
Was test control completed to verify results?			
Were contaminated items discarded correctly?			
Were test results accurately recorded?			

Evaluator:____________________________ Date:______________

Suggestions for Improvement:____________________________

Procedure Evaluation Form

NAME:____________________

PROCEDURE:____________________

Technique	Yes	No	Comments
Were Standard Precautions followed?			
Was equipment prepared correctly?			
Were the procedural steps properly followed?			
Was test control completed to verify results?			
Were contaminated items discarded correctly?			
Were test results accurately recorded?			

Evaluator:____________________ Date:__________

Suggestions for improvement:____________________

Procedure Evaluation Form

NAME:____________________

PROCEDURE:____________________

Technique	Yes	No	Comments
Were Standard Precautions followed?			
Was equipment prepared correctly?			
Were the procedural steps properly followed?			
Was test control completed to verify results?			
Were contaminated items discarded correctly?			
Were test results accurately recorded?			

Evaluator:____________________ Date:__________

Suggestions for improvement:____________________

UNIT VI MICROBIOLOGY

CHAPTER 23 INTRODUCTION TO MICROBIOLOGY

MATCHING

Match the terms in the right column with the definitions in the left column by writing the letters in the blanks.

	Definition	Term
_____	1. Organization the produces guidelines for the handling of biohazardous waste in the lab.	a. Autoclave
_____	2. The ratio of sick to well people in a community.	b. Epidemic
_____	3. Decontaminates air of infectious material.	c. Nosocomial
_____	4. Ratio of total number of deaths to the total population.	d. Morbidity
_____	5. Organization that provides labels for biohazard materials.	e. Contagious disease
_____	6. A sterilizing instrument that uses steam at high pressure.	f. OSHA
_____	7. Refers to infection starting inside the hospital.	g. Sodium hypochlorite
_____	8. Can be spread by direct or indirect contact.	h. HEPA
_____	9. An effective agent against viral contamination.	i. CDC
_____	10. Widespread occurrence of disease among many people in a given region at the same time.	j. Mortality

SHORT ANSWER

Answer the following questions:

11. Identify the ways by which microorganisms can contaminate a specimen.

____

____

____

12. List the procedure steps for proper packaging of a specimen for transport out of your area.

____

____

____

13. Compare and contrast a laboratory cabinet and a biological safety cabinet.

____

____

14. How can air containing infectious materials be decontaminated?

____

____

____

15. Site the probable points of origin for exposure to microorganisms in the medical office.

____

____

____

CRITICAL THINKING

Decide how you would handle the following situations, using the knowledge you have obtained in this chapter, combined with previously learned knowledge.

Situation #1

While moving a rack of culture tubes to the autoclave area, you drop the entire rack, causing most of the tubes to shatter and the contents to spill onto the floor. You are responsible for cleaning up the biohazardous spill.

1. Site the Standard Precaution regulations that determine the method of cleanup.

____

____

____

2. List the apparel that you will need to wear during the cleaning process.

____

____

____

3. Identify the equipment that you will use to decontaminate the area.

____

____

4. Will you need to report the accident and/or file an incident report? Why?

____

____

CHAPTER 24 SMEAR PREPARATION, STAINING TECHNIQUES, AND WET MOUNTS

MATCHING

Match the terms in the right column with the definitions in the left column by writing the letters in the blanks.

_____ 1. Filaments or threads composing the mycelium of a fungus	a. Morphology
_____ 2. A substance that fixes a stain or dye.	b. Media
_____ 3. A microorganism having a long whip-like, mobile appendage.	c. Spores
_____ 4. Spherical bacteria.	d. Hyphae
_____ 5. A nutritive substance upon which bacteria will grow.	e. KOH mount
_____ 6. Rod bacteria.	f. India ink
_____ 7. Study of the form and structure of organisms, tissues, and cells.	g. Cocci
_____ 8. Refractile, oval bodies formed within bacteria.	h. Flagellates
_____ 9. Helpful when examining samples for fungal elements.	i. Mordant
_____10. Used for direct visualization of encapsulated yeast.	j. Bacilli

SHORT ANSWERS

Answer the following questions:

11. Describe how the Gram stain is used in identifying bacteria.

____

____

____

12. A smear can be made from the following body sites.

____

____

____

13. Describe proper technique for staining bacteria.

____

____

____

14. Describe the microscopic appearance of:

Cocci ____________________

Bacilli ____________________

Spirillum ____________________

15. Using brightfield microscopy or phase-contrast microscopy, specimens can be applied directly to the surface of a slide for immediate examination. Identify the organisms that are best visualized by:

Direct saline mount:____________________

Potassium hydroxide mount:____________________

India ink preparation:____________________

CRITICAL THINKING

Decide how you would handle the following situations, using the knowledge you have obtained in this chapter, combined with previously learned knowledge.

Situation #1

Ms. S was diagnosed with *Trichomonas vaginalis*. What type of sample was most likely used to confirm her diagnosis? Explain the laboratory testing technique. Identify the causative organism.

____

____

____

____

Situation #2

Today the laboratory receives a new shipment of media for bacterial cultures. How would you handle the shipment and where would it be stored until it is needed? If you have never done this before, what would be your strategy to ensure that you do it correctly?

____

____

____

Procedure Evaluation Form

NAME:____

PROCEDURE:____

Technique	Yes	No	Comments
Were Standard Precautions followed?			
Was equipment prepared correctly?			
Were the procedural steps properly followed?			
Was test control completed to verify results?			
Were contaminated items discarded correctly?			
Were test results accurately recorded?			

Evaluator:______________________________ Date:_______________

Suggestions for improvement:______________________________

Procedure Evaluation Form

NAME:____

PROCEDURE:____

Technique	Yes	No	Comments
Were Standard Precautions followed?			
Was equipment prepared correctly?			
Were the procedural steps properly followed?			
Was test control completed to verify results?			
Were contaminated items discarded correctly?			
Were test results accurately recorded?			

Evaluator:______________________________ Date:_______________

Suggestions for improvement:______________________________

CHAPTER 25 CULTURE TECHNIQUES

MATCHING

Match the terms in the right column with the definitions in the left column by writing the letters in the blanks.

Definition	Term
_____ 1. Pus in the urine.	j. Bacilli
_____ 2. Air intolerant.	b. Pyuria
_____ 3. Show best growth in oxygen.	c. Lyse
_____ 4. Allows nonfastidious organisms to grow at their natural rates.	d. Bacteriuria
_____ 5. Bacteria in the urine.	e. Aerobic
_____ 6. Antibacterial substance used in treating a wide range of infections.	f. Glomerulonephritis
_____ 7. Destruction of cells or cell contents.	g. Endocarditis
_____ 8. Inflammation found in the kidney.	h. Hemolytic
_____ 9. Inflammation of the lining of the heart and heart valves.	i. Anaerobic
_____10. Pertaining to the rupture of erythrocytes and the release of hemoglobin into plasma.	j. Bacitracin

SHORT ANSWER

Answer the following questions:

11. List guidelines you must follow when collecting and transporting specimens.

____

____

____

12. Why do anaerobic specimens require special handling? How is this achieved?

____

____

____

13. Identify the environmental conditions that have an effect on bacterial growth.

____

____

____

14. Give four examples of culture media.

____________________ ____________________

____________________ ____________________

15. Identify the media you would use to culture suspected:

Enteric bacilli:____________________

Routine throat cultures:____________________

Gonorrhea:____________________

Skin ulcer exudates:____________________

Urinary tract infection: ____________________

16. Identify the two species that represent the majority of isolates seen in urine cultures.

____________________ ____________________

17. Explain the process of semiquantitative streaking.

____

____

____

18 Explain the process for obtaining a throat swab sample for culture.

____

____

____

CRITICAL THINKING

Decide how you would handle the following situations, using the knowledge you have obtained in this chapter, combined with previously learned knowledge.

Situation #1

Ms. T has been instructed to bring a first morning voided urine specimen into the office for culturing. When she arrives at the office, the waiting room is full of people. She is embarrassed to bring the sample to the appointment window, so she leaves it with the test request on the floor of the waiting room. At about 10:00 AM the package is noticed, retrieved, and sent to the laboratory for testing.

1. Can this sample be used or should it be rejected? Why?

2. Why would pyuria be an important finding in regard to her diagnosis?

Situation #2

Mr. G returns to the office with open sores on his lower legs, which the physician diagnosed as leg ulcers due to poor circulation and long-standing diabetes mellitus. The physician requests a culture and sensitivity to determine if staphylococcus is the infecting organism.

1. How would you obtain the sample?

2. Describe the technique you would use to make and stain the culture and the smear?

3. How would you prepare the culture for microscopic examination?

4. If this is positive for *Staphylococcus aureus*, what would you expect to see under the microscope?

Procedure Evaluation Form

NAME:____

PROCEDURE:____________________________________

Technique	Yes	No	Comments
Were Standard Precautions followed?			
Was equipment prepared correctly?			
Were the procedural steps properly followed?			
Was test control completed to verify results?			
Were contaminated items discarded correctly?			
Were test results accurately recorded?			

Evaluator:______________________________ Date:______________

Suggestions for improvement:______________________________

Procedure Evaluation Form

NAME:____

PROCEDURE:____________________________________

Technique	Yes	No	Comments
Were Standard Precautions followed?			
Was equipment prepared correctly?			
Were the procedural steps properly followed?			
Was test control completed to verify results?			
Were contaminated items discarded correctly?			
Were test results accurately recorded?			

Evaluator:______________________________ Date:______________

Suggestions for improvement:______________________________

CHAPTER 26 BACTERIOLOGY

MATCHING

Match the terms in the right column with the definitions in the left column by writing the letters in the blanks.

_____ 1. Normally harmless species of bacteria that has become pathogenic under specific circumstances.

_____ 2. A parasitic organism that causes no harm to the host.

_____ 3. Formation of discharge of pus.

_____ 4. Morphological changes indicative of enzymatic cell death.

_____ 5. An infection acquired during hospitalization.

_____ 6. Gram-positive cocci that grows in clusters

_____ 7. An enzyme that causes coagulation of citrated plasma.

_____ 8. Gram-positive cocci that grow in chains.

_____ 9. Diffuse inflammatory process within solid tissue.

_____ 10. Inflammation in the folds of tissue surrounding the nail.

a. Necrosis
b. Commensal
c. Suppuration
d. Paronychia
e. Nosocomial
f. Staphylococcus
g. Streptococcus
h. Cellulitis
i. Opportunistic
j. Coagulase

SHORT ANSWER

Answer the following questions:

11. What are the four standard factors used for identifying bacteria in the lab?

____

____

____

____

12. Identify the four basic bacteria groups.

____

____

____

____

13. *Streptococcus pyogenes* is frequently the pathogenic agent in what common illnesses?

____

____

____

14. Explain the "Camp Factor".

____

____

____

15. What syndrome is identified with the outbreak of *E.Coli* associated with fast food burgers.

____

16. Tuberculosis infections seem to be spreading. Identify the geographical areas and the groups of people showing the highest incident rate.

____

____

17. Describe catalase and how it is used.

____

____

____

18. The Spot-indole test characterizes what bacteria? How does color indicate results?

____

____

19. List the four ways in which bacteria are produced in the gastrointestinal tract.

____

____

____

____

20. What bacterial infections can be encountered concurrent with a burn wound?

____

____

CRITICAL THINKING

Decide how you would handle the following situations, using the knowledge you have obtained in this chapter, combined with previously learned knowledge.

Situation #1

Mrs. J.J. is a seven-day post-op abdominal hysterectomy patient. She has a definite foul-smelling drainage oozing from her incision. The physician orders a culture and sensitivity of the drainage.

1. How would you obtain the culture?

   ____

2. What isolation media would you select to use for the culture? Why?

   ____

3. After the incubation period, the growth is prepared for viewing. Under the microscope you see Gram-positive cocci in definite clusters. They appear to be a creamy white color, large in size, and higher in the middle than around the edges. The light from the scope does not appear to shine through the growth. What type of organisms do you suspect have been isolated?

   ____

4. After the lab tech has completed the analysis, you are instructed to clean up the area and are told to discard the culture. How will you do this?

   ____

   ____

Situation #2

During a pelvic examination, Ms. L's gynecologist notices bleeding at the cervix. He obtains a genital swab of the area and orders laboratory testing to determine the causative organism. He writes on the Lab request "R/O chlamydia".

1. What tests should be done on the sample?

   ____

2. If his diagnosis is correct, what would you expect to see on the culture plate and under the microscope?

   ____

   ____

Procedure Evaluation Form

NAME:____________________

PROCEDURE:____________________

Technique	Yes	No	Comments
Were Standard Precautions followed?			
Was equipment prepared correctly?			
Were the procedural steps properly followed?			
Was test control completed to verify results?			
Were contaminated items discarded correctly?			
Were test results accurately recorded?			

Evaluator:____________________ Date:__________

Suggestions for improvement:____________________

Procedure Evaluation Form

NAME:____________________

PROCEDURE:____________________

Technique	Yes	No	Comments
Were Standard Precautions followed?			
Was equipment prepared correctly?			
Were the procedural steps properly followed?			
Was test control completed to verify results?			
Were contaminated items discarded correctly?			
Were test results accurately recorded?			

Evaluator:____________________ Date:__________

Suggestions for improvement:____________________

CHAPTER 27 BASIC MYCOLOGY, PARASITOLOGY AND VIROLOGY

MATCHING

Match the terms in the right column with the definitions in the left column by writing the letters in the blanks.

_____ 1. Jock itch.	a. Dermatophytid
_____ 2. Ringworm.	b. Hyphae
_____ 3. A subkingdom of unicellular organisms that are frequently ingested and transmitted through contaminated feces.	c. Tinea corporis
	d. Mycobacterium
_____ 4. A slender, acid-fast microorganism resembling the bacillus that causes tuberculosis.	e. Tinea cruris
	f. Protozoan
_____ 5. A phylum of the animal kingdom that includes arachnids, crustaceans, and insects.	g. Tropozoite
	h. Oocyst
_____ 6. The active, motile feeding stage of a protozoan parasite.	i. Endemic
_____ 7. A secondary skin eruption occurring on an area remote from the site of infection.	j. Arthropods
_____ 8. Filaments or threads composing the mycelium of a fungus.	
_____ 9. Present in a community at all times.	
_____10. Analogous stage in the development of any sporozoan.	

SHORT ANSWER

Answer the following questions:

11. Name and describe two forms of dimorphic fungi.

____

____

12. What are the symptoms of tinea pedis and what laboratory test is used to confirm the diagnosis?

____

____

____

13. What is *Coccidioides immitis* and why is it endemic?

____

____

14. List the human symptoms of enterocolitis and how this diagnosis is confirmed.

____

____

15. Name and describe three common diagnostic tests used to identify a fungal disease.

____

____

____

16. Describe the ways by which parasites are transmitted.

____

____

____

____

17. Identify the three groups of parasitic worms.

____

____

____

18. List five of the most common viruses.

____________________ ____________________

____________________ ____________________

____

19. Describe the different manifestations of the herpesvirus.

____

____

20. The 'chronic carrier' occurs in which hepatitis virus?

____

What does this term mean?

____

CRITICAL THINKING

Decide how you would handle the following situations, using the knowledge you have obtained in this chapter, combined with previously learned knowledge.

Situation #1

Mr. P presents with complaints of diarrhea and fatigue. After examination, it is found that he is also suffering from intestinal bleeding. He reports that he has been living in unsanitary conditions in South America.

1. What is a possible cause for his condition?

____

____

2. The physician asks you to check on the tests that need to be run and where the samples would have to be sent to determine the causative pathogen. Where would you look for this information?

____

____

3. When you find the location of the closest laboratory that can handle the testing required, you call the laboratory. What information do you need to obtain from this reference laboratory?

____

____

____

Situation #2

Mr. C owns a large chicken ranch near Cleveland Ohio. He has a positive skin test for Histoplasmosis.The physician is not alarmed at this finding and tells Mr. C not to worry about the positive skin test unless he develops other symptoms.

1. What type of symptoms should Mr. C be advised to watch for?

____

____

2. Why is the physician not alarmed at the positive results to the test done on Mr. C?

____

____

Procedure Evaluation Form

NAME:________________________________

PROCEDURE:________________________________

Technique	Yes	No	Comments
Were sSandard Precautions followed?			
Was equipment prepared correctly?			
Were the procedural steps properly followed?			
Was test control completed to verify results?			
Were contaminated items discarded correctly?			
Were test results accurately recorded?			

Evaluator:____________________ Date:__________

Suggestions for improvement:____________________

Procedure Evaluation Form

NAME:________________________________

PROCEDURE:________________________________

Technique	Yes	No	Comments
Were Standard Precautions followed?			
Was equipment prepared correctly?			
Were the procedural steps properly followed?			
Was test control completed to verify results?			
Were contaminated items discarded correctly?			
Were test results accurately recorded?			

Evaluator:____________________ Date:__________

Suggestions for improvement:____________________

UNIT VII MEDICOLEGAL ISSUES

CHAPTER 28 ANCILLARY RESPONSIBILITIES

MATCHING

Match the terms in the right column with the definitions in the left column by writing the letters in the blanks.

_____ 1. Study of the formation, structure, function, biochemistry, and pathology of the cells.

_____ 2. The process of cell division that results in the formation of two daughter cells and the replacement of dead cells.

_____ 3. The study of disease.

_____ 4. The process of two cells fusing into one cell, which may result in the formation of a zygote.

_____ 5. Study of the distribution and conditions of disease in a defined population.

_____ 6. The study of origin, structure, function, and pathology of tissue.

_____ 7. Disease attacking many people in a region at the same time.

_____ 8. Makes up cell walls and cell membranes.

_____ 9. Animal that transfers pathogenic organisms.

_____10. Science that deals with cause of disease.

a. Mitosis
b. Meiosis
c. Pathology
d. Vector
e. Epidemiology
f. Phospholipids
g. Epidemic
h. Cytology
i. Etiology
j. Histology

SHORT ANSWER

Answer the following questions:

11. Describe the two types of infections in which epidemiology is concerned.

____

____

12. What are the three epidemiological factors concerning susceptibility of disease?

____

____

____

13. Identify the three primary reasons why new infectious agents continue to arise.

____

____

____

14. List the six principle causative factors that describe diseases.

______________ ______________

______________ ______________

______________ ______________

15. List ten well-known communicable diseases.

______________ ______________

______________ ______________

______________ ______________

______________ ______________

______________ ______________

16. List four diseases that you have studied that are caused by vectors.

______________ ______________

______________ ______________

17. Compare the processes of meiosis and mitosis.

____

____

18. Identify two histology techniques ?

____

____

Explain these two procedures.

____

____

____

____

19. What is a microtome and how is it used?

____

____

CRITICAL THINKING

Decide how you would handle the following situations, using the knowledge you have obtained in this chapter, combined with previously learned knowledge.

Situation #1

In the past year, everyone working in your office complex has had repeated upper respiratory infections. There have been several who have had throat cultures done with results being positive for strep. Management has stated that if you have a fever, you are not to come to work but that hasn't stopped the problem.

1. What do you think is the problem?

____

____

____

2. List the steps that should be followed to isolate the cause.

____

____

____

3. Should this be reported to the local public health office? Why?

____

____

____

____

4. Could you be the problem? Justify your self-defense.

____

____

____

Situation #2

A family member has a tumor removed surgically. After the operation is completed the surgeon comes into the waiting room and tells the family that the tumor was not cancerous, it was benign, and there is nothing to worry about. How was the surgeon able to do this tissue analysis so quickly? It usually takes 24-72 hours to get the results of a laboratory test.

Visit a local hospital laboratory and ask if you can interview the histologist or the individual that is responsible for tissue biopsy specimens. Report on the procedural technique that makes this analysis possible in just minutes.

____

____

____

____

____

____

____

Procedure Evaluation Form

NAME:____

PROCEDURE:____

Technique	Yes	No	Comments
Were Standard Precautions followed?			
Was equipment prepared correctly?			
Were the procedural steps properly followed?			
Was test control completed to verify results?			
Were contaminated items discarded correctly?			
Were test results accurately recorded?			

Evaluator:____ Date:__________________

Suggestions for improvement:____

Procedure Evaluation Form

NAME:____

PROCEDURE:____

Technique	Yes	No	Comments
Were Standard Precautions followed?			
Was equipment prepared correctly?			
Were the procedural steps properly followed?			
Was test control completed to verify results?			
Were contaminated items discarded correctly?			
Were test results accurately recorded?			

Evaluator:______________________________ Date:________________

Suggestions for improvement:______________________________

CHAPTER 29 FORENSIC PATHOLOGY

MATCHING

Match the terms in the right column with the definitions in the left column by writing the letters in the blanks.

_____	1. The stiffening of fibers of all muscles.	a. Livor mortis
_____	2. Cooling of the body.	b. Cadaveric spasm
_____	3. The discoloration by gravitation of blood.	c. Rigor mortis
_____	4. Violent spasm of muscles at time of death.	d. Algor mortis
_____	5. An anatomical elevated structure of the skin, usually more than 5 mm in diameter.	e. Asphyxia
		f. Unnatural
_____	6. Occurring in the ordinary course of events.	g. Forensic
_____	7. Deficiency of oxygen and increase of carbon dioxide in the blood and tissues.	h. Bleb
		i. Unnatural
_____	8. Pertains to legal proceedings and elements of law.	j. Pathology
_____	9. Branch of medicine dealing with the essential nature of disease.	
_____	10. Not in accordance with the usual physical nature of a person.	

SHORT ANSWER

Answer the following questions:

11. Define " unnatural deaths" as it pertains to forensic medicine. Cite examples.

____

____

____

12. What must be determined before a death certificate can be issued?

____

____

Who issues the death certificate?

____

13. What factors determine the agency responsible for a death investigation?

14. What kinds of physical evidence are recorded during the police investigation?

15. Compare the two types of autopsy examination.

16. What is time of death based on?

17. When do blebs occur? Explain this phenomena.

.18. What is the usual order of decomposition in the body?

19. When are entomologists called in during an investigation?

20. What does dry heat prevent?

CRITICAL THINKING

Decide how you would handle the following situations, using the knowledge you have obtained in this chapter, combined with previously learned knowledge.

Situation #1

A coroner arrives on the scene of a death. The body is noted to exhibit a bright, cherry red staining of the skin. It is consistent with what level of deterioration and can be contributed with what type of death?

1. What type of autopsy determination is this?

   ____

   ____

2. Who will be responsible for the death certificate?

   ____

   ____

3. In your home county, can the family of the deceased refuse to allow an autopsy?

   ____

   ____

CHAPTER 30 LEGAL ISSUES

MATCHING

Match the terms in the right column with the definitions in the left column by writing the letters in the blanks.

_____ 1. Indirect legal responsibility of an employer for the wrongful act of an employee.

_____ 2. Doctrine by which the one who sells a defective product is responsible for damages.

_____ 3. Doctrine applied when relationship between master and servant (employer/employee) exists at the time of wrongdoing.

_____ 4. Civil wrong or injury other than breach of contract for which the court will provide an action for damages.

_____ 5. Enforces guideline for Universal Precautions.

_____ 6. When a person did or did not do something that a reasonable person would have done or not done in similar circumstances.

_____ 7. Established guidelines for Universal Precautions.

_____ 8. Reasonable anticipation that harm or injury is a likely result of acts or omissions.

_____ 9. Prohibits discrimination against disabled persons.

_____10. Facts that give a person the right to judicial relief.

a. Strictly liable
b. Tort
c. Respondeat superior
d. CDC
e. Negligence
f. Vicariously liable
g. OSHA
h. Cause of action
i. Foreseeability
j. ADA

SHORT ANSWER

Answer the following questions:

11. List the four elements necessary for a cause of action for negligence.

____

____

____

____

12. Name the four conditions that must be satisfied for the doctrine of Res ipsa loquitur to be applied.

____

____

____

____

13. List the eight targeted classifications of discrimination.

____________________ ____________________ ____________________

____________________ ____________________ ____________________

____________________ ____________________

14. The ADA prohibits discrimination against ______________________________.

15. Identify three hazards, associated with technology, that laboratory personnel face.

____

____

____

16. Define "intentional tort" and give an example that applies to the laboratory.

____

____

____

17. Identify the two Occupational Safety and Health Act obligations imposed on employers.

____

____

18. Are infractions of the Act ever considered criminal? Justify your answer with examples.

____

____

____

19. Define sexual harassment in your own words.

____

____

____

20. What is the most important step you can take to prevent sexual harassment?

____

____

____

CRITICAL THINKING

Decide how you would handle the following situations, using the knowledge you have obtained in this chapter, combined with previously learned knowledge.

Situation #1

Mrs. O goes into the lunch room to eat and in the room are four men from radiology, eating. They are talking about a comedy film that one of them rented over the weekend. Mrs. O sits down and begins to eat her lunch and the men continue their conversation. The man that rented the film repeats a very sexist joke that was on the film and the other three begin laughing and making comments about the joke. Mrs. O packs up her remaining lunch and leaves the room, never speaking to any of the men. The following week each of the four men and the medical office receive a court summons for sexual harassment charges against Mrs. O.

1. Under what conditions is the employer/company liable?

____

____

2. Do you feel that Mrs. O has a justifiable case? Why?

____

____

3. Looking at the law, what section is her attorney using to establish a case?

____

____

4. What section of the law would the defense attorney use?

____

____

Situation #2

Ms. K has filed a suit against a laboratory, claiming that a deep thrombosis in her arm was caused by a deep jab of the phlebotomist's needle as he obtained an arterial blood sample.. She claims she was stabbed so hard she flinched, causing the needle to penetrate her arm too deeply. The defendant claims the patient refused to have her arm strapped to the table, which is his usual mode of operation when obtaining an arterial blood sample. He further states that she did jerk but he hit the artery and obtained the sample on the first attempt.

1. What conditions of Res ipsa loquitor are met?

____

____

2. What conditions of this Doctrine are not in this case?

____

____

3. Knowing arterial draws are painful, what could have been done to ward off the chance of litigation?

____

____

____

____

ANSWER KEY

UNIT I

Chapter 1

Matching
1. C
2. E
3. B
4. A
5. D

Short Answer
6. Collect adequate blood specimens by correct method
   Correctly label all specimens
   Start glucose tolerance procedures
   Perform automated testing
   Assist, as directed by supervisor, in testing procedures
7. Physician's offices, HMO, clinics, private reference labs, public health departments
8. Biochemical properties of an organism
   Growth patterns of cultured microorganisms
   Sensitivity of an organism to antibiotics
9. Chemistry, microbiology section, serology, serology, microbiology, microbiology, hematology, pathology, serology, anatomic pathology lab, serology

Critical Thinking
Situation #1 answers will vary
Situation #2 answers will vary

Chapter 2

Matching
1. D
2. H
3. G
4. C
5. J
6. I
7. B
8. F
9. A
10. E

Short Answer

11. high voltage, flammable solvents, toxic chemicals, bio-hazardous waste
12. chain of infection-cross contamination of infectious waste
13. reservoir host--means of transmission--means of entry--new host
14. blood vessels at site dilate- WBC in area increase-redness
    WBC consumes pathogens-Phagocytosis
    fluid in injured tissues increases-edema
    increased blood supply to the area-heat
15. Hepatitis A; most common form-viral
    Hepatitis B; serum hepatitis; 10% become chronic carriers
    Hepatitis C; known as non-A non-B; debilitating symptoms
    Hepatitis D; known as delta virus; causes illness only in HBV infected persons
    Hepatitis E; enteric hepatitis; caused by consuming contaminated food and water
16. engineering-biosafety cabinets, autoclaves
    personal protection-gloves, gowns (masks, eye protection)
    work practice-cleaning and disposal of needles
    lab specimens-handling specimens, cleaning spills
    infectious waste-removal of waste, decontamination of lab

Critical Thinking

Situation #1 answers will vary

Situation#2

1. break in communication
2. refusal form-print out discussing immunization and answering questions
3. ask her to come to the office to discuss concerns

Chapter 3

Matching

1. B
2. D
3. E
4. A
5. C

Short Answer

6. Quality Assurance-a set of policies and procedures developed to ensure quality
   Quality Control-application of methods and means to ensure reliable, valid results
7. POL-simple screening and automated tests
   commercial-CLIA regulations, 3 categories of tsting complexity
8. Complete laboratory inventory
   CLIA and OSHA guidelines to ensure QA program, exists for all tests
   Register the POL with the HCFA

Documentation system including all steps taken in lab testing
Organize precise QC program including every test done in lab
Apply for certification

Critical Thinking
Situation #1 Documentation must follow manufacturers testing protocols
Situation #2 Out of date supplies

Chapter 4

Matching
1. D
2. F
3. E
4. G
5. I
6. H
7. B
8. C
9. J
10. A

Short Answer
11. bright field
12. very small bacteria such as spirochete
13. living prokaryotic and eukaryotic microorganisms
14. fluorescence microscope
15. electron beam instead of visible light
    magnets instead of lenses
    dry specimen mounted in wax or plastic-direct visualization

Critical Thinking
Situation #1 compare with lab maintenance manual
Situation #2 uses no visible light or lens
human eye has nothing to focus on

Chapter 5

Matching
1. D
2. E
3. H
4. J

5. I
6. C
7. G
8. B
9. F
10. A

Short Answer
11. kilometer
12. cubic centimeter
13. maintaining the standards upon which this system is based
14. ampere, kilogram, second, candela, meter, mole, kelvin
15. decimals

Critical Thinking
Situation #1 kilo
hecto
deca
meter
deci
centi
milli
micro
nano
Situation #2 soda, liquor, cough syrup, metric sockets and wrenches, sporting events (races)

Chapter 6

Matching
1. E
2. H
3. F
4. I
5. J
6. D
7. C
8. A
9. B
10. G

Short Answer
11. quantity, consistency, color, odor, transparency, sediment, froth

12. dark red, bean-shaped, 10-12 cm. long, 5-6 cm. wide, 2.5 cm. thick, weight 8oz., located retroperitoneal
13. one million of them consisting of renal corpuscle, glomerulus, Bowman's capsule
14. to detect body disturbances and to detect intrinsic conditions that may adversely affect the kidneys and urinary tract
15. identify patient
    record the time the specimen was voided
    time specimen was centrifuged
    final testing time
    chart the results

Critical Thinking

Situation #1 the most frequently encountered lab errors involve testing the wrong specimen or recording the results on the wrong chart

Situation #2 answers will vary

UNIT II

Chapter 7

Matching

1. H
2. G
3. B
4. C
5. I
6. E
7. F
8. J
9. D
10. A

Short Answer

11. Carefully label all specimen containers, not the container lids
    Provide a precleaned or sterile container that will hold 50 to 100 mL and has an opening of 2 inches in diameter.
    For bacterial culture make sure container is sterile.
    Female patients should avoid collecting urine specimens during menstrual period.
    It analyte is unstable or testing is delayed add preservative to the specimen.
12. Answers may vary
13. Be sure the specimen is thoroughly mixed , and quantity is measured and recorded. Prepare a representative sample for transport. Follow the recommended procedure of the laboratory that will be conducting the test.

14. Neonate=20-350 mL/24 hr
    Child (1-9 yrs) = 300-600 mL/24 hr
    Adolescent (10-16 yrs) = 600-1500 mL/24 hr
    Adult= 600-2000 mL/24 hr
15. Premoistened towelettes, a sterile specimen container, and illustrated instructions.

Critical Thinking

Situation #1 Type=clean-catch specimen. Commercial kit containing the items llisted in #15. Instructions described in figure 7-4 for both female and male.

Situation #2 Urine should be tested immediately if this is not possible the specimen should be refrigerated. If left at room temperature the chemistry of the sample will change and the results will be false.

Chapter 8

Matching

1. F
2. H
3. I
4. E
5. A
6. C
7. B
8. D
9. J
10. G

Short Answer

11. Hematuria- Hemoglobinuria- Porphyrins- Blood- Bilirubin
12. The kidney's ability to concentrate and dilute urine.
13. pH=diet, medication, and disease
    Glucose=diabetes mellitus
    Ketone= incomplete fat metabolism,diabetes mellitus
    Protein= see table 8
    Blood= infectious diseases, trauma, neoplasms
    Bilirubin= viral hepatitis, obstructive disease
    Urobilinogen= intestinal disease, obstructive bilirubin disease
    Nitrite= enteric gram-negative bacteria, bacteria in urine
    Leukocyte esterase= Urinary tract infections, bacteriuria
14. Use brightfield microscope; examine unstained or stained with supravital stain. Polarized microscopy useful in identification of crystals. Phase-contrast improves visibility of translucent material.
15. Compare with Figs 13, 14, 15, and 16.

Critical Thinking
Situation #1
1. Diabetes mellitus
2. No, test used was specific for glucose only.
3. Detectable levels of ketone may occur in urine in physiological stress conditions such as diabetes mellitus, fasting, pregnancy, or strenuous exercise.
4. Complications include nephropathy, glomerulus becomes converted into an eosinophilic hyaline mass, chronic renal failure, necrosis of the glomeruli, and death

Situation #2
1. Protein and oval fat bodies; Normally no protein is detectable in urine, although minute amounts may be secreted by the kidneys. Oval fat bodiesare frequently found with nephrotic syndrome and with an elevated protein.
2. Glomerulonephritis or nephrotic syndrome
3. Sulfasalocylic acid, Bence Jones

Chapter 9

Matching
1. A
2. J
3. H
4. A
5. C
6. B
7. F
8. G
9. E
10. D

Short Answer
11. Once the placenta begins to form, it secretes hCG which spills into the urine.
12. Urine + anti hCG inhibits the latex beads so that there is no binding with the anti hCG, thus blocking the patient's hCG.
13. Quantity measures the amount which is excreted over a 24-hour period.
14. Elevated urinary excretion. Tests include black or ultraviolet light as porphyrins fluoresce.
15. Easy obtained, drug concentrations are typically higher, urine drug levels may remain elevated when drug is no longer detected in the blood.

Critical Thinking
Situation #1
1. Intact RBC's in urine may give urine a red color with cloudy appearance. These RBC's are visable upon microscopic exam. Lysed or destroyed RBC's may give the urine a pink or red color with a clear appearance. No RBC's would be seen in the microscopic exam. This

seems to correlate with the microscopic finding however, you should have a positive finding for blood on the reagent strip in either case. There was no such finding in this patient.
2. Specimen has been altered in some way by the patient. Possible workers compensation fraud which is a felony.

Situation #2
1. Abnormal dark yellow, cloudy, 3+ blood, > RBC
2. Kidney stones
3. Repeat urinalysis, intravenous urography

UNIT III

Chapter 10

Matching
1. I
2. D
3. E
4. G
5. J
6. A
7. H
8. C
9. F
10. B

Short Answer
11. Granulocytes:
    1. basophils-contain heparin and histamine for clotting and allergic responses
    2. eosinophils-engulf substances that trigger allergies
    3. neutrophils-accumulate at infection site and engulf and destroy bacteria and debris

    Agranuloytes:
    1. lymphocytes-attack foreign matter and make antibodies which neutralize and destroy antigens
    2. monocytes-crawl into tissue at infection site where they surround and eat agents causing the infection
12. anemia, thrombocytopenia, thrombocytosis, polycythemia, leukemia (etc)
13. Platelets form from giant multinucleated cells, called megakaryocytes, from which they break off in fragments. Their main function is to help blood coagulate.
14. occurs in hematopoietic tissue of red bone marrow, lymph nodes, spleen, thymus and GI tract
15. answers may vary

Critical Thinking

Situation #1

1. See Figure 10-1
2. Activation of the body's defense mechanism.
3. Infection or invasion of foreign matter and activation of the body's immune system.

Situation #2

1. Allergy or immune disorders
2. Radioallergosorbent test (RAST)
   Radio immunoassay (RIA)
   Fluorescent antibody techniques
   Agglutination tests
   Precipitation
   Sensitivity

Chapter 11

Matching

1. G
2. J
3. I
4. H
5. A
6. B
7. C
8. D
9. E
10. F

Short Answer

11. select the proper venipuncture method
    prepare patient for the procedure
    perform venipuncture and specimen collection
    observe puncture site before releasing patient
12. when attempting to draw from infants, small children, or adults with difficult veins
13. heparin and EDTA;
14. when veins are very small or fragile; invert to mix, then label appropriately
15. patient name, chart # or date of birth, time of collection, test(s) ordered,
    date and phlebotomist's initials; after tube contains blood and has been mixed

Critical Thinking

Situation #1

1. Remove the needle from the patient's arm and place apply pressure to the puncture site.
   Notify your supervisor, take the patient's pulse and blood pressure.

2. Put him in a supine position before drawing. Ask him if he would prefer to come in tomorrow morning for the draw.

Situation #2

1. Have only the supplies that are needed on the tray and cover these with a drape until you need them. Have a book or game for Child to look at while you prepare to draw. Obtain the blood sample as quickly as possible, with as little discussion as possible. Save talking for after the draw is completed.
2. Butterfly with syringe-less traumatizing due to small veins and fear of procedure.
3. Have mother hold the child and assist in securing the arm at the time of the draw. If mother can not do this, ask a colleague to assist you.

Chapter 12

Matching

1. I
2. J
3. A
4. G
5. H
6. B
7. C
8. F
9. D
10. E

Short Answer

11. RBC count, RBC morphology, RBC indices, WBC count, differential WBC count, platelet count, platelet morphology, hemoglobin determination, hematocrit determination
12. *aplastic-abuse to the stem cells in bone marrow by toxic substances.
    *Folate acid deficiency-decreased folate acid level from alcohol, liver disease, acute leukemia, ulcerative colitis and infantile hyperthyroidism.
    *hemolytic anemia-destruction of red blood cells.
    *iron deficiency-blood loss through hemorrhage, chronic loss from hemmorroids, ulcer and menorrhea.
    *pernicious anemia-lack of B12 due to inadequate absorption in GI system.
    *sickle cell-abnormal form of hemoglobin (hemoglobin S).
13. cyanmethemoglobin, hemoglobinometer, specific gravity method
14. MCV, MCH, MCHC
15. polycythemia vera
    anemia
    polycythemia vera
    anemia
    Improper collection or processing techniques

Critical Thinking

Situation #1

MCV=84 fL   MCH= 30 pg   MCHC= 35.7 g/dL

Situation #2

The tube must sit in the vertical position, tilting the tube will cause an increase in ESR reading. undisturbed for one hour. If it is jarred, bumped, or moved during the testing period, the test results may be invalid as vibration may increase ESR results. Both Mark and Scott are in the wrong.

Chapter 13

Matching

1. G
2. H
3. F
4. B
5. I
6. D
7. J
8. A
9. C
10. E

Short Answer

11. Factor XII makes contact with damaged vessel surfaces and activatesthe intrinsic pathways. This reation results in stimulation of the common pathway. Factor XII is released when tissue damage occurs. It, along with Factor V stimulates common pathway and fibrin clot occurs.
12. It is an inherited sex-linked recessive gene caried on X chromosome
13. between 5-10 minutes;
14. prothrombin time-between 11-14 seconds
    partial thromboplastin-30-45 seconds
    activated coagulation time-70-120 seconds
15. the time taken for a standardized skin wound to stop bleeding
16. Ivy bleeding time-between one and eight and a half seconds
17. Tilt tube method was performed for manual coagulation studies. Small test tubes were tilted at timed intervals until the first appearance of clot.
18. Heparin cannot be taken orally and coumadin can be. Anticoagulation is almost immediate after heparin is given. Coumadin is used for long term maintenance. Protime and/or PPT would be used to monitor the affects of Coumadin. PT or PTT tests are ordered before and during therapy with optimal results being 1.5 to 2.5 times the control value.

Critical Thinking

Situation #1

1. Yes it may altar the clotting mechanism
2. Notify your supervisor or call and report this to the physician and/or hospital admitting.

Situation #2

1. Check the laboratory procedure manual for guidelines on warming blood for a stat protime. Follow the recommendations. If you cannot locate the needed guidelines, check with your supervisor as to how you should proceed with this test. If the test cannot be completed, call the physician before 5:00 PM and explain the circumstances.

UNIT IV

Chapter 14

Matching

1. J
2. G
3. F
4. I
5. H
6. A
7. B
8. D
9. C
10. E

Short Answer

11. 1 liter graduated cylinder
    50-100 ml graduated cylinder
    pH paper, urine collection containers (3L for 24 hr collection, 4oz routine)
12. a. 60-105 mg/dL
    b. 2.7-8.5 mg/dL
    c. 3.5-5.0 mEq/L
    d. 4-18 mg/dL
    e. 2.7-8.5 mg/dL
13. 4 degrees C
14. -20 degrees C
15. 2000-3500 rpm
16. speed, plasma may be processed immediately
17. It must be collected anaerobically.
18. They are to be considered infectious and guidelines for Universal Precautions must be observed.
19. To indicate normal and abnormal tests

20. Prepare collection container by adding sodium bicarbonate and cover container with foil. Pour aliquot of specimen in. When instructing patient, tell them to discard the first morning specimen on day one and record the time. Collect all specimens during the remaining day and night. Collect first morning specimen day 2 at the exact time first morning specimen was discarded. Make sure label has all patient information and starting and ending times.

Critical Thinking

Situation #1 Check with a local reference laboratory or hospital laboratory.

Situation #2 Your draw would depend on the type of chem panel ordered. Page 187 in the text lists possible tube combinations. The turbid appearance can indicate improper collection or handling of the sample or a disease state of the patient.

Chapter 15

Matching

1. E
2. J
3. H
4. B
5. A
6. C
7. I
8. F
9. D
10. G

Short Answer

11. (any five)
    colorimetric
    spectrophotometry
    kinetic method
    enzymatic method
    Ion specific method
    Flame photometry
    atomic absorption
12. volumetric- used when accurate transfer of volume is critical
    graduated-used for measuring different volumes
    Pasteur-used to add small unmeasured quantities to receptacles
13. a. BUN 10 milligrams in a deciliter
    b. 103 milliequivalents per liter
    c. uric acid 5.7 milligrams in a deciliter

14. Ion specific electrode(ISE)- each electrode has properties of permeability which are specific for only one ion. The sample is entered into the system and flows through, interacting with the elctrode membrane, diffuses through the interface, creating an impulse. The impulse is measured and processed by the instrument.
15. volumetric pippettes are used for exact measure whereas the graduated is used for non-critical measure

Critical Thinking

Situation #1

See Table 15-1, page 201 in your text and the index for reference ranges.

Situation #2

25 mL of hcl + 475 mL of H_2O= 500 mL of 5% hcl solution

Chapter 16

Matching

1. G
2. J
3. A
4. F
5. B
6. I
7. D
8. H
9. E
10. C

Short Answer

11. (choose any four)
    alkaline phosphatase (ALP)
    serum glutamic-pyruvic transaminase (SGPT)
    aspartate transaminase (AST)
    serum glutamic oxaloacetic transaminase (SGOT)
    gamma-glutamlytransterase (GGT) -tested on a lab chemistry analyzer
12. An elevated level of either can indicate MI, especially if CPK elevates before LDH

Critical Thinking

Situation #1

A. hypercholesterolemia

B. gout

C. diabetes mellitus

D. acute renal failure

E. hepatic disorder, multiple sclerosis

Situation #2
1. 2.6 RF
2. 3.1 RF
3. Patient 2

Chapter 17

Matching
1. C
2. A
3. J
4. E
5. D
6. I
7. H
8. F
9. B
10. G

Short Answer
11. The same results is obtained when the speimen is analyzed by mutliple methods.
12. latex agglutination, radioimmunoassay, fluorescence polarization immunassay, EMIT
13. organophosphate pesticide poisoning (Malathion)
14. iron, arsenic, mercury and lead; iron and lead
15. ethanol
16. isopropanal (rubbing alcohol)
17. paranoid psychoses
18. cocaine
19. opium
20. general anesthesia, pain relief, glaucoma treatment, chemotherapy side effects (nausea, vomiting)

Critical Thinking
Situation #1 Mr. O as urine output positive for alcohol can represent uncontrolled diabetes
Situation #2 Check with your supervisor and/or the office protocol manual for instructions. Usually this is noted on the laboratory request form and the patient is instructed to obtain a medstream sample or the requesting physician may order a catheterized sample.

Chapter 18

Matching
1. C
2. F
3. J
4. B
5. H
6. I
7. A
8. G
9. E
10. D

Short Answer
11. *know the dosage size, form and means of administration
*must have compliance of dosage regimen
*must know the time of the last dose of medication prior to blood sampling
*must record blood sample time
*blood sample must be drawn at optimal time for the drug being tested

12. *minimum effective range (MEC) and minimum inhibitory concentration (MIC)
*bacteriostatic antibiotics and sulfonamides
*steady state peak concentrations-Amoxil
*maximum to minimum steady staate concentration-gentamycin
*mean state-digoxin
*therapeutic window-Diazepam
13. Any time, at least six hours after the dose.
See Fig. 18-11
14. Answers will vary
15. Appropriately stocked phlebotomy tray, timing device, appropriate requisition and laboratory forms.

Critical Thinking
Situation #1 Trough level sample is drawn immediately prior next dose =6:55 or 12:55. The peak level sample is drawn at 7:55 or 1:55. Refer to Procedure 18-1 in text.
Situation #2 J. B.= within therapeutic range
S.B.= slightly elevated but not markedly
L.L.= toxic level exceeded, immediate action required
A.B.= marked low response, report to supervisor/physician.

Chapter 19

Matching
1. B
2. I
3. A
4. G
5. J
6. H
7. F
8. E
9. C
10. D

Short Answer
11. The fluorescent anti-nuclear antibody detects the presence of antinucleoprotein factors, amongst the many complicated antibodies, by forming identifiable patterns that are associated with the disease
12. Patient antigen and known amount of labeled antigen are mixed with a specific antibody. Bound and free substances are separated by charcoal absorption, salt or solvent precipitation, solid phase antibody or double antibody techniques. The amount of patient antigen is based on a determination of either the free or the bound labeled antigen. Standard curve is used to quantify patients antigen.
13. the number of dissolved particles in a solution; electrolyte balance and maintenance of homeostasis
14. First-ABO blood group type
    Second-MN blood group system and Rh
    Lastly-Human leukocyte antigen (HLA)
15. PSA antigen is found in both normal prostatic cells and prostatic cancer cells, PAP is not

Critical Thinking
Situation #1 They are identical twins
Situation #2
1. Refer to Table 19-4
2. Test should be rerun due to low oxygen content, high carbon dioxide content, and skewed base excess and deficit.

UNIT V

Chapter 20

Matching

1. C
2. J
3. E
4. F
5. A
6. D
7. H
8. I
9. G
10. B

Short Answer

11. Active immunity is acquired over a long period of time and protects the body against new infections as a result of antibodies that develop naturally or artificially. Passive immunity is acquired from the antibodies transferred through the placenta to the fetus or through the colostrum to the infant or artificially by vaccination/immunization.
12. B cells and T cells. B cells originate in the bone marrow and migrate to lymphatic tissue. It can transform into an antibody-producing plasma cell. T-cells are stored in the thymus gland and are the body's memory cells of immunity. Both cells work in body defense against invading pathogens.
13. IgG as it forms antibodies and activates complement.
14. Blood banking is concerned with antibody screening and compatibility testing.
15. Large phagocytes that destroy worn-out RBC, and clear away other dead cells and debris caused by infection.

Critical Thinking

Situation #1 Active immunity as a result of antibodies forming naturally over a long period of time.

Situation #2 This antigen will create antibodies as a result of the injection of the antiserum in a program of prophylactic therapy.

Chapter 21

Matching

1. D
2. H
3. J

4. B
5. F
6. A
7. C
8. E
9. G
10. I

Short Answer

11. Bioluminescence-chemiluminescence; hormones
    ELISA; AIDS and Hepatitis A and B
    Agglutination; brucella, salmonella
    RIA precipitation; bacterial exotoxins, fungi
    Compliment Fixation; VDRL(syphillis)
    Neutralization; viral infections
    Fluroescent Antibody-syphillis
12. A false positive test result indicates a test reaction that identifies a patient who who does not have the condition of disease in question but tests positive
13. determination of titer by diluting the specimen being tested and performing the serological test in question on each dilution
14. The incubated known virus and test serum are inoculated into the tissue and the effects noted. The test serum is given and the test animal is challenged with microorganisms. If antibody is present in the test serum, the animal is protected against infection

Critical Thinking

Situation #1 Rheumatoid arthritis. Tests could include slide agglutination techniques such as Seratest RF Latex Kit, and RF Latex Test.

Situation #2 Answers will vary depending on methods employed.

Chapter 22

Matching

1. G
2. D
3. B
4. I
5. F
6. J
7. C
8. H
9. A
10. E

Short Answer

11. *prevent transfusion and transplant reactions
    *identify the potential for hemolytic disease of newborn
    *determine parentage
    *forensic purposes
12. type A, type B, type AB, type O
13. When D antigen is present, agglutination occurs when anti-D antiserum is reacted with RBC's; if D antigen is not present, no agglutination will occur. Patients with Rh positive blood will agglutinate in the presence of anti-D serum but not with the control. Patients with Rh negative blood will NOT agglutinate in the presence of anti-D nor the control
14. Rh negative patients transfused with blood from Rh positive donor or blood of Rh positive fetus passes through the placenta and enters the circulatory system of Rh negative mother
15. mental retardation, stunted growth or death
16. high titer anti-Rh gamma globulin
17. chills, fever, headache, hives, burning sensation
18. *blood group and type
    *reaction of recipient's with donor's (compatability)
    *antibody screen

Critical Thinking

Situation #1 Type A or Type B could be used as there would only be one type of antibodies opposing in either one. In Type O there would be both A and B antibodies.

Situation #2

1. Autologous
2. A+, A-, O+, or O-.
3. There are no antigens on cells of Type O blood making it possible to use the packed cells as universal donation.
4. Antibody B

Situation #3

1. Blood group=A
2. Positive (+)
3. See Figure 22-6 in text
4. Antibody=B

UNIT VI

Chapter 23

Matching

1. F
2. D

3. H
4. J
5. I
6. A
7. C
8. E
9. G
10. B

Short Answer

11. *bacteria from patient's normal bacterial flora
    *by person collecting specimen
    *from environment
    *introducing unwanted organism into specimen
12. Specimen collected in a special vial or tube preferably with an unbreakable plastic or glass inner core. Seal tube with special tape to prevent leakage and then place in larger outer container of metal or plastic with a leak proof lid and packed with absorbent material. Then, insert into cardboard mailing carton, seal and labeled appropriately.
13. biosafety cabinets encase a work area, protecting lab personnel from exposure to infectious diseases
14. through HEPA air filter or exposure to UV light or heat
15. Any object or structure that is touched or handles by staff or patients is a probable point of origin. The more the exposure the greater the exposure.

Critical Thinking

Situation #1

1. Refer to Chapter 2 in the text.
2. Barrier gown, gloves, face protection, and shoe protection (if you have to step into the contaminated substance).
3. One commerical biohazardous clean-up and disposal Kit. Use Procedure 23-2 for guidelines.
4. Yes, all accidents regardless of their cause, nature, or outcome, must be reported. Many insurance providers will want a copy for their files.

Chapter 24

Matching

1. D
2. I
3. H
4. G
5. B

6. J
7. A
8. C
9. E
10. F

Short Answer

11. Bacteria stains either gram positive (deep violet) or gram negative (red); gram positive bacteria is not affected by alcohol, so does not decolorize from the violet color, but gram negative bacteria is damaged and causes the violet iodine complex to leak out leaving a red color identification
12. any body opening including genital or wounds
13. apply a sequence of primary stain, mordant, decolorizer and counterstain; for fixed smear, place onstaining rack, pour primary stain on one end until whole slide is covered and allow to remain for 30 secs.; decant and rinse
14. spherical; rod, oval-like; rigid spirials, corkscrew
15. trichomonas vaginalis; fungal elements; encapsulated yeast

Critical Thinking

Situation #1 Vaginal secretions and/or vaginal mucus. Wet mount usually a direct saline mount is the testing techniques. Causative organism =*Trichomonas vaginalis.*

Situation #2 First check the protocol manual for specific instructions used for each of the media received. Follow these instructions . If there are no protocols to cover this procedure, read themanufacturer's instructions that are enclosed with each group of media and follow these instructions. If this cannot be located, contact your supervisor for instructions. Remember to always rotate older media forward and place the new behind so that the oldest gets used first This eliminates the problem with expired media that cannot be used.

Chapter 25

Matching

1. B
2. I
3. E
4. A
5. D
6. J
7. C
8. F
9. G
10. H

Short Answer

11. *specimen should be collected in the area most likely to produce the suspected microorganism with as little contamination as possible
    *specimen quantity should be sufficient to permit the required exams
    *specimen should be placed in designated sterile containers
    *closer to the onset of disease, the greater the likelihood that the causative microorganism will be isolated
    *whenever possible, specimens for microbiological exams should be collected before administration of antimicrobial agents
    *specimens should be promptly transported to lab for testing
    *specimens improperly collected or transported may be rejected; follow rejection guidelines carefully and explain to the physicin ordering
12. They are air-intolerant. Use an air tight container to preserve integrity of sample.
13. temperature, moisture, nutrients, Ph and salt concentration
14. (choose four) blood agar, chocolate agar, MacConkey agar, SSA, chopped meat broth, Thayer Martin agar, HE
15. Enteric bacilli=MacConkey agar
    Routine throat cultures=SSA
    Gonorrhea=chocolate agar
    Skin ulcer excudates=blood agar
    Urinary tract infections= blood agar
16. *E.Coli* and *Staph*
17. An innoculating loop, calibrated to retain .001 ml of urine, is immersed into an uncentrifuged urine sample and a streak is made across the center of an agar plate. The inoculum is then diluted by spreading evenly at right angles to the primary streak. Resterilize the loop between each phase of streaking. Label the agar side of dish with patients name, date, time and type of specimen used. Place sample into incubator, agar side up and incubate 18-24 hours. Count colonies of bacteria.
18. While holding the tongue down with a depressor, take specimen from back of throat and tonsils with a sterile Dacron swab in a lazy 8 pattern. Avoid teeth and inside of mouth. Use two swabs and place in sterile tube with media if its a culture. Label tube appropriately.

Critical Thinking

Situation #1

1. Sample should be rejected as it was not refrigerated and since it was on the floor, unattended, it cannot be verified as belonging to the patient.
2. It would confirm or rule out possible infectious pathogens present.

Situation #2

1. Use a sterile collection tube, making sure it was correctly labeled. Remove samples of fluid and exudates from the ulcerative site and place it in the sterile collection tube for transport.
2. Follow same technique as used in Procedure 24-1 and 24-2

3. Follow same technique as used in Procedure 24-3
4. See figure 24-10

Chapter 26

Matching
1. I
2. B
3. C
4. A
5. E
6. F
7. J
8. G
9. H
10. D

Short Answer

11. cellular morphology, colony morphology, biochemical testing and antibiotic sensitivity testing
12. gram positive cocci, gram negative cocci, gram positive bacilli, gram negative bacilli
13. cellulitis, tonsillitis, pharyngitis, otitis media, bronchopneumonia, rheumatic fever, acute glomerulonephritis, septicemia and meningitis
14. camp factor is a compound that acts in concert with the beta toxin produced by certain strains of S. Aureus to create enhanced beta hemolysis.
15. hemolytic-uremic syndrome (HUS)
16. spreading in large cities and effecting elderly, noncaucasians, alcoholics, AIDS patients and health care workers
17. Catalase is a rapid enzyme test used to distinguish members of the genus streptococcus from those of staphylococcus.
18. Spot-indol is used to characterize E. coli and resulting color is blue-green
19. *by producing toxin
    *causing loss of function through the destruction of the intestinal mucosa
    *through invasion and destruction of the mucosal epithelium causing septicemia
    *through invasion of the intestional mucosa thereby interfering with absorption and secretion
20. various *Streptococci, S. aureus*, S. *epidermidis*, *Enterobacteriaceae pseudomonas*, and other gram negative bacilli

Critical Thinking
Situation #1
1. Follow procedure used in Chapter 26, Situation #2 in the workbook

2. Blood agar as it allows determination of whether an organism is hemolytic.
3. *Candida albicans*
4. Following laboratory protocols for biohazardous waste. This is usually autoclaving of the specimen to render it harmless.

Situation #2

1. Cell culture, DNA probes, and immunoassay; See Procedure 26-5 in text
2. See Figure 26-12 and 27-22 in text.

Chapter 27

Matching

1. E
2. C
3. F
4. D
5. J
6. G
7. A
8. B
9. I
10. H

Short Answer

11. molds and yeast
12. itching, scaling, or blisters containing thin watery fluid on soles of feeet or between toes; KOH mount
13. San Joaquin Valley Fever found in Kern County all the time
14. low grade fever, watery or mucous diarrhea, persistant gastroenteritis with vomiting and abdominal cramping and malabsoption; identified by oocyst in fecal sample
15. *direct microscpic exam of tissue scrappings
    *Wood's light
    *KOH mount
16. *ingestion of infective stage
    *direct penetration of skin by infective larvae
    *inoculation by an arthropd vector
17. *nematodes, or roundworms
    *cestodes, or tapeworm
    *trematodes, or flukes
18. measles, herpes, mononucleosis, mumps, influenza, chicken pox, HIV, AIDS, hepatitis
19. herpes simplex, herpes zoster, genital herpes
20. Hepatitis B; capable of spreading the disease to others for an indefinite period of time

Critical Thinking
Situation #1
1. Amoebic dysentery
2. Look in the Laboratory protocol manual for reference laboratory that tests for *Entamoeba hystolytica*. If you are unable to find the name of a reference laboratory, call the laboratory that does the physician's routine microbiology analysis and ask for a referral laboratory.
3. The type of sample(s) required, how to collect the sample, method of preparation, and method of transport, and method of billing including cost.

Situation #2
1. Mild respiratory illness to temporary incapacity with general malaise, weakness, fever, chest pains, and a dry or productive cough.
2. He lives in the major endemic area and he is exposed to bird droppings every day. He is not showing any signs of illness.

UNIT VII

Chapter 28

Matching
1. H
2. A
3. C
4. B
5. E
6. J
7. G
8. F
9. D
10. I

Short Answer
11. community acquired and nosocomial
12. *susceptibility of patient
    *virulence of infecting organism
    *nature of exposure
13. *changing lifestyles of people
    *travel of people carrying communicable disease
    *biological emergence of new infectious bacteria and viruses
14. heredity, infectious organisms, life-style, accidents, poisons and toxic chemicals
15. cold, measles, mumps, gonnorhea, tuberculosis, small pox, typhoid fever, diphtheria, tetanus, whooping cough
16. malaria, rabies, typhus, ringworm
17. meiosis-two cells fuse into one (formation of zygote)

mitosis-when one cell divides to make two cells

18. specimen collection, tissue processing and analysis
19. specimen collected by surgical biopsy using different types of specialized needles; specimen is then sent to a pathologist to be examined. Processing includes fixation, dehydration, cleaning and infiltration. It is then embedded in melted paraffin and once hardened, processed in a microtome.
20. A microtome is a specialized instrument used to cut tissue samples for microscopic examination. It cuts wax-embedded sample into 1-inch thick sections so that ir can be fixed on glass slides and stained

Critical Thinking

Situation #1

1. Nosocomial infection
2. Everyone in the office should have a throat culture, urine culture, and a stool culture to discover who is the carrier.
3. Yes, due to the nature of the business and the possible patient exposure
4. Answers will vary

Situation #2

1. Individual report on findings.

Chapter 29

Matching

1. C
2. D
3. A
4. B
5. H
6. F
7. E
8. G
9. J
10. I

Short Answer

11. not in accordance with the usual physical nature of a person; asphyxia, suffocation, strangulation, suicide, homicide (etc)
12. cause and manner of death; coroner's office or medical examiner
13. where death occurred and circumstances surrounding it
14. blood stains, photographs, fingerprints, position of deceased, type of injuries, possible instruments used and other crime paraphenalia
15. external-overall investigation of physical body including wounds, injuries, traumatized areas, r/o sexual assault or molestation, etc

internal-exam of internal organs including weight, measurement, gross description and samples of tissue analysis

16. cadaveric spasm, rigor mortis, algor mortis, livor mortis, decomposition, insect activity and putrefaction
17. occur during decomposition; when cells break down, anaerobic gas-forming organisms move into systemic vein where small bubbles disrupt the tissue causing the 'blebs'
18. *intestines, stomach, liver, blood, heart muscle
    *lungs
    *brain
    *kidneys, bladder and testes
    *voluntary muscle
    *uterus and prostate
19. when a body is discovered partially decomposed and there is overwhelming fly activity
20. bacterial decomposition and putrefaction

Critical Thinking

Situation #1 Level of deterioration=Livor mortis Type of death= unnatural

1. Forensic
2. County coroner or medical examiner
3. Answers will vary depending upon living location

Chapter 30

Matching

1. F
2. A
3. C
4. B
5. G
6. E
7. D
8. I
9. J
10. H

Short Answer

11. duty to use reasonable care; breach of this duty by failure to comply with regular standard of care; a reasonably close factual and legal connection between the negligent conduct and resulting injury; actual injury, damage or loss to another
12. Event doesn't normally occur unless someone is negligent; caused by an agent or instrument totally within the defendant's control; event is not due to any

voluntary action by the plaintiff; evidence of the true explanation of event is more readily accessible to the defendant than the plaintiff

13. age, sex, race, color, creed, marital status, national origin or disabilities
14. disabled
15. musculoskeletal, such as CTS, vision problems due to constant computer screen use, stress related illnesses
16. the intentional civil wrong or injury done to another for which the court will provide a remedy in form of an action for damages; a patient forced to have a blood draw against their will
17. provide employment free of recognized hazards and comply with Safety and Health Standards Act
18. Yes, examples will vary
19. answer will vary
20. education and training as well as investigating claims of harassment thoroughly and complete documentation.

Critical Thinking

Situation #1

1. Conduct within the office is under the employers liability.
2. Answers will vary
3. Title VII sex-based discrimination
4. Act was not deliberate and the conversation was not directed at her. The employer was not aware of act. Defendant did not tell the men that their conversation was to stop as she found their comments to be sexually discriminate.

Situation #2

1. The burden of proof rests on the defendant. The four conditions to satisfy the doctrine are met verbally. See page 418 in text.
2. What was documented. We have no knowledge of the written evidence.
3. Patient education prior to the procedure. An informed patient is more cooperative.